Springer
Tokyo
Berlin
Heidelberg
New York
Barcelona
Budapest
Hong Kong
London
Milan
Paris
Singapore

H. Ishikura (Editor-in-Chief)
M. Aikawa, H. Itakura, K. Kikuchi
(Editors)

Host Response to International Parasitic Zoonoses

With 64 Figures, Including 38 in Color

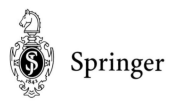

Springer

Editor-in-Chief:
HAJIME ISHIKURA, M.D.
Professor, Division of Parasitology, Department of Pathology
Sapporo Medical University School of Medicine
Minami 1, Nishi 17, Chuo-ku, Sapporo 060-8556, Japan

Editors:
MASAMICHI AIKAWA, M.D., Ph.D.
Professor, Research Institute of Medical Sciences, Tokai University
Bohseidai, Isehara, Kanagawa 259–1193, Japan

HIDEYO ITAKURA, M.D., Ph.D.
Professor, Department of Pathology, Institute of Tropical Medicine
Nagasaki University, 1-12-4 Sakamoto, Nagasaki 852-8523, Japan

KOKICHI KIKUCHI, M.D., Ph.D.
Department of Pathology, Sapporo Medical University School of Medicine
Minami 1, Nishi 17, Chuo-ku, Sapporo 060-8556, Japan

ISBN 4-431-70217-2 Springer-Verlag Tokyo Berlin Heidelberg New York

Library of Congress Cataloging-in-Publication Data
Host response to international parasitic zoonoses / H. Ishikura,
    editor-in-chief ; M. Aikawa, H. Itakura, K. Kikuchi, editors.
        p.   cm.
    Includes bibliographical references and index.
    ISBN 4-431-70217-2 (hardcover : alk. paper)
    1. Zoonoses—Histopathology—Congresses.   2. Zoonoses—Diagnosis—
Congresses.   3. Zoonoses— Epidemiology—Congresses.   4. Medical
geography—Congresses.   5. Host-parasite relationships—Congresses.
I. Ishikura, H. (Hajime), 1915–   .
    [DNLM: 1. Zoonoses congresses.   2. Host-Parasite Relations
congresses.   3. Parasites—pathogenicity congresses.   WC 950 H831
1998]
RC113.5.H67   1998
616.9′59—dc21
DNLM/DLC
for Library of Congress   98-21933

Printed on acid-free paper

© Springer-Verlag Tokyo 1998

Printed in Hong Kong

Typesetting, printing, & binding: Best-set Typesetter Ltd., Hong Kong
SPIN: 10656049

Preface

At its 86th annual meeting, the Japanese Pathological Society decided to conduct a symposium on the subject of the pathology of international parasitic zoonoses. It was somewhat unusual for the Japanese Pathological Society to organize a symposium on parasitology. However, recent trends in parasitic diseases in Japan had made pathologists aware of the dual necessity for commitment to parasitology and for opportunities to discuss the pathology of globalized parasitic diseases.

With increased internationalization of food and lifestyles, Japanese pathologists and clinicians now have more knowledge than ever about imported parasitic diseases such as malaria, amebic dysentery, and cutaneous leishmaniosis, and about the global spread of parasitic diseases such as anisakidosis and *Diphyllobothrium nihonkaiense* infection. In addition, Japanese pathologists and clinicians need extensive, up-to-date knowledge of the worldwide status of parasitic diseases so as to help to control those diseases in underdeveloped countries where parasites are still a major cause of death. However, there is a tendency for Japanese medical schools to close their departments of parasitology, converting them to departments that are concerned with other new and sophisticated fields of research. Among 85 medical schools in Japan, 22.0% in 1987 and 23.8% in 1997 did not have departments of parasitology. Pathologists thus are required to seek out more opportunities to teach students about new trends in parasitology and to diagnose new parasitic diseases among patients.

The symposium was held in Sapporo in June 1997 and was well received by the participants. Topics of discussion included parasitology and international health, the pathology of parasitic zoonoses, recent trends and pathology of imported parasites, new methodology to diagnose parasitic diseases, and molecular technology to detect and diagnose parasites.

This monograph includes the contents of the symposium along with additional material on important current problems in parasitic diseases from a global point of view. We hope that this book will help the reader to achieve a better awareness and understanding of the interactions between human beings and pathologic parasites in the 21st century.

October 1997
HAJIME ISHIKURA
KOKICHI KIKUCHI

Table of Contents

Pathology and Differential Diagnoses of Internationalized Zoonoses: Summarizing Discussion of the Organizers

Hajime Ishikura[1], Masamichi Aikawa[2], and Hideyo Itakura[3]

This chapter presents a summary of eight lectures of Symposium 6 of the 86th Annual Meeting of the Japanese Society of Pathology, held in Sapporo, Japan, June 4–6, 1997. Pathological aspects of parasitic diseases and related topics were discussed in the symposium, including host-to-parasite relationships and imported parasitic disorders. Pathological, diagnostic, and preventive topics of imported zoonoses were vigorously discussed. The discussions concerning these important problems were very much appreciated by the members of the Japanese Society of Pathology.

The symposium first addressed issues on international relationships between Japan and other countries, such as those in Southeast Asia, Central Africa, and Middle and Southern America. Japan gives aid to these countries in the form of Japanese educational parasitologists and sends volunteers, mainly through the organizations of Official Development Assistance (ODA) and the Japan International Cooperation Agency (JICA).

Diphyllobothrium nihonkaiense has been identified as a novel parasite by a collaboration of Japanese and Finnish parasitologists. Possible human diseases caused through infection by this worm could have important implications. According to Yamane, who spoke on this topic, parasites responsible for diphyllobothriosis found in Japan from 1982 to 1995 included *Diphyllobothrium latum* (1560 cases), *D. nihonkaiense* (57), *D. yonagoense* (17), *D. pacificum* (6), *D. cameron* (1), *D. hians* (1), *D.*

[1] Division of Parasitic Diseases, Department of Pathology, Sapporo Medical University School of Medicine, Minami 1, Nishi 17, Chuo-ku, Sapporo 060-8556, Japan
[2] Research Institute of Medical Sciences, Tokai University, Bohseidai, Isehara, Kanagawa, 259-1193, Japan
[3] Department of Pathology, Institute of Tropical Medicine, Nagasaki University, 1-12-4 Sakamoto, Nagasaki 852-8523, Japan

scoticum (1), *D. orcini* (1), *D. erinacei* (adult, 12), *Diplogonoporus grandi* (19), and *Diphyllobothrium fukuokaense* (1). He also reported that a total of 1855 cases of diphyllobothriosis were found in Japan during this period. Table 1 shows that 124 of 231 worms (53.4%) of the genus *Diphyllobothrium* reported in Asahikawa and Okayama were suspected to be *D. nihonkaiense*. Yamane also stated that 57 of the 1855 cases (3%) were *D. nihonkaiense*, which allows us to make the following estimation from a statistical point of view: as our patients with diphyllobothriosis numbered 230, 7 cases could have been caused by *D. nihonkaiense*. In the remaining 223 patients, diseases appeared to be related to infection by *D. latum*, *D. yonagoense*, *D. pacificum*, *D. cameron*, *D. hians*, *D. scoticum*, *D. orcini*, *Spirometra erinacei* (adult), *Diplogonoporus grandi*, and *Diphyllobothrium fukuokaense*. Similar disorders have been found, caused by hitherto unidentified species of the genus *Diphyllobothrium*, which possibly harbor in marine mammals that migrate seasonally in the sea around Japan. Yamane summarized the important international problems into the following four categories: (1) clarification of the distinction between *D. nihonkaiense* reported in Japan and *D. klebanovskii* in Russia; (2) clarification between *D. nihonkaiense* in Japan and *D. laum* in Korea; (3) issues on synonyms, especially in relation to infection sources; and (4) the urgent need to establish intimate global collaboration among parasitologists all over the world.

The next speaker, Dr. Nawa, stressed the need for mass screening of humans and animals from a preventive point of view. He also described detailed procedures of identification of causative worms from feces or sputum. He noted that, in combination with examination for blood eosinophilia, helminth-specific diagnoses were possible by a combined use of multiple-dot enzyme-lmked immunosorbent assay (ELISA), a double-immunodiffusion test in agarose gel, and binding-inhibition tests of micro-ELISA methods. By using these combined methods, he obtained a highly specific diagnosis among populations in the northern Kyushu area. He addressed the urgent need to become familiar with identification of parasite eggs, as well as with hematoxylin-eosin diagnosis, and this included a recommendation of high-power observation of parasites by pathologists.

Dr. Aikawa, who has 40 years of experience studying parasitic disease at Case Western Reserve University (Cleveland, OH, USA), gave a presentation on the pathology of cerebral malaria. Malaria was the most widespread disease in the world up to 1995. Therefore, Japanese travelers

Table 1. Doubtful cases of *Diphyllobothriosis nihonkaiense*[a]

Case no.	Name	Report year	Classification name	Area	No. of cases	Remarks
1.	T. Kihara et al.	1973	– Doubtful	Okayama	14	
2.	Y. Yazaki et al.	1983	– D. latum	Asahikawa	9	Double
3.	Y. Yamane et al.	1986	+ nihonkaiense	Shimane		Double
4.	M. Tada et al.	1990	– Doubtful	Kyoto	3	
5.	A. Nakayoshi et al.	1990	+ nihonkaiense	Okinawa	4	
6.	M. Ozaki et al.	1990	+ nihonkaiense	Tokyo	10	
7.	T. Taya et al.	1990	– Failure	Asahikawa	43	
8.	T. Ebe et al.	1990	+ Doubtful	Tokyo	8	
9.	J. Maejima et al.	1991	+ D. yonagoenses	Tottori	13	Another
			D. pacificum			
			D. cameroni		46	
			D. hians			
			Diphyllobothrium sp.			
10.	T. Mori	1991	+ D. latum	Tokyo	1	Another
11.	J. Maejima et al.	1991	+ nihonkaiense	Tottori	4	
12.	T. Fukushima et al.	1991	+ D. latum	Shimane		Another
			D. dendriticum		(animal experiment)	
13.	R. Ito et al.	1991	– Doubtful	Akita	4	
14.	S. Nishikawa et al.	1992	– Doubtful	Hyogo	3	
15.	S. Fukumoto et al.	1992	+ D. yonagoense	Kyushu	2	Another
16.	T. Matsuura et al.	1992	+ nihonkaiense	Shinshu	0	

Table 1. *Continued*

Case no.	Name	Report year	Classification name	Area	No. of cases	Remarks
17.	T. Harada et al.	1992	− *Doubtful*	Niigata	2	
18.	K. Sugi et al.	1993	+ *nihonkaiense*	Osaka-Kyoto	6	
19.	Y. Iwata et al.	1993	+ *nihonkaiense*	Gunma	2	
20.	Y. Yamane et al.	1993	+ *nihonkaiense*	Shimane	12	
21.	M. Hagino et al.	1994	− Failure	Fukui	41	
22.	S. Yamaguchi et al.	1994	− Doubtful	Tokyo	2	
23.	K. Ohnishi et al.	1994	+ *nihonkaiense*	Tokyo	1	
24.	N. Nishiyama et al.	1995	+ *nihonkaiense*	Nara	1	
25.	M. Endo et al.	1995	− Failure	Tokyo	1	
26.	K. Sugawara et al.	1996	− Doubtful	Tokyo	1	
27.	R. Yanagisawa et al.	1996	+ *nihonkaiense*	Tokyo	1	
28.	N. Takayama et al.	1996	+ *nihonkaiense*	Tokyo	4	
29.	H. Hoshino et al.	1996	− Doubtful	Kanagawa	2	
30.	S. Hokama et al.	1996	− Doubtful	Okinawa	3	
				Total	231	

[a] Summary:

Doubtful, failure	124
D. nihonkaiense	45
D. latum	1
D. yonagoense	15
D. pacificum, D. cameron, D. hians, Diphyllobothrium sp.	46
Total	231

sometimes become infected with the disease abroad, after which they eventually become ill in Japan. Tropical malaria is accompanied by a high death rate because of its tendency to progress to cerebral malaria. Human erythrocytes infected by malaria express cellular adhesion molecules at the knob on the surface of cell membranes that subsequently attach to endothelial cells in the brain through specific attachment between adhesion molecules, including occlusion of blood vessels and bleeding. Occlusion appears also in the heart and other organs, thus leading to the death of the patient. An effective vaccine or antimalaria therapy must be developed in the near future through an understanding of this mechanism.

Dr. Tsutsumi, using many beautiful histological slides that were typical and diagnostic for individual diseases, presented data on pathological findings of host response which are useful for the routine diagnostic activity undertaken by pathologists. The parasitic diseases he presented included amebiosis, toxoplasmosis, cryptosporidiosis, and cutaneous leishmaniosis. Although immunohistochemical identification of parasite-specific antigens is critical in diagnosis, antibodies specific to these antigens are not commercially available at the present time. His most successful attempt has been utilization of patients' sera in their recovery phase. Sera were used as primary antibodies for indirect immunoperoxidase staining, using formalin-fixed, paraffin-embedded materials. Demonstrations given of antigens reactive with patients' sera at the disease sites were impressive.

By use of enzyme multifocus electrophoresis, Lia Paggi from Italy presented her data on anisakid phenotypes, which have been accepted by parasitologists worldwide. She introduced her current data on molecular genetics in anisakid nematodes from the Pacific Boreal region. Siblings of Anisakidae captured in Japan were also discussed. Previously studied worms. *Anisakis simplex* sensu lato, L3, *Pseudoterranova decipiens* sensu lato, L3, *Contracaecum osculatum* sensu lato, adult, and intermediate hosts caught in several different places in Hokkaido were first discussed. The sibling search revealed that *A. simplex* sensu stricto in Hokkaido was related to *P. bulbosa* and *P. azarasi*, and that *Contracaecum osculatum* in Hokkaido was the C. D. type. A detailed phenotypic analysis of the variety of worms was reported by her, and these findings have been accepted by parasitologists all over the world.

Takahashi et al. summarized anisakidosis, based on these data and an exploration of the literature, an updated analysis of which revealed that there have been 30 000 or more cases of anisakidosis in Japan, while there have only been 1000 or fewer outside Japan. He discussed these data and stated that the Japanese custom of eating raw fish in the form of sushi, sashimi, or battera is responsible for the outstandingly great incidence of the disease in this country. He also estimated that anisakidosis cases that had not been reported in Japan could put the total at as many as 100 000 cases. In addition, cases outside Japan are increasing rapidly, apparently because of the gradual growth in popularity of Japanese food in other countries.

Takahashi showed a detailed analysis of intermediate host species and anisakid species, revealing a relationship between the spatial distribution of these species and disease forms. He stated that pseudoterranovosis predominated in Hokkaido because marine mammals are infested by adult *Pseudoterranova* worms, and emphasis was placed on infection of humans by adult *Pseudoterranova*. This indicates that *Pseudoterranova* larvae infected and grew in humans, and this appears to be a hitherto unknown relationship between the human host and anisakid parasites. Morphological differentials among *Anisakis*, *Pseudoterranova*, *Hysterothylacium aduncum*, and *Porrocaecum reticulatum* were briefly discussed. Species of parasites, intermediate fish hosts, and sea mammals, and their distribution and proliferation, have been greatly influenced by global weather and pollution. This problem was discussed in combination with examples such as El Niño and CO_2 pollution.

Acknowledgments and Conclusions

We thank Professor Kokichi Kikuchi, Department of Pathology, Sapporo Medical University School of Medicine, for giving us the opportunity to discuss many important aspects of parasitological problems with members of the Japanese Society of Pathology. We also thank the members of the Society, as many as 500, who participated in the discussion for 3 h. We believe that this symposium could help pathologists become familiar with parasitic diseases and help them to make easier diagnosis of these diseases when encountered. This symposium will be followed by a symposium at the 9th International Congress of Parasitology to be held in 1998 in Makuhari, Chiba. A Contracaecum Forum will be held in Sapporo in late August or early September in 1998, where Drs. Paggi from Italy, Berland of Norway, Fagerhorm of Finland, and four additional Japanese speakers are presenting their data. Some of the data on anisakisosis and anisakids are now available on the Internet at "Anisakis 110-ban," where information about these issues is open to the public.

References

Ebe T, Matsumura M, Mori T, Takahashi M, Kohara T, Inagaki M, Isonuma H, Hibiya I, Hamamoto T, Funayama H, Ikemoto H (1990) Eight cases of *Diphyllobothriosis*. J Jpn Assoc Infect Dis 64:328–334 (in Japanese)

Endo M, Matsuhisa T (1995) An experience of *Diphyllobothriosis latum* removed by gastrografin. Clin Parasitol 6:66–68 (in Japanese)

Fukumoto S, Maejima J, Yazaki S, Hirai K, Tada I, Yamamoto S (1992) The two cases of *Diphyllobothrium yonagoense* in the Kyushu district—revision and indentification of previously reported cases. Jpn J Parasitol 42:16–23 (in Japanese with English abstract)

Fukushima T, Abe K, Isobe A, Shiwaku K, Yamane Y, Bylund G (1991) The comparative histological observations on the effects of antihelmintics to *Diphyllobothriid cestodes*. Jpn J Parasitol 40(suppl):123 (in Japanese)

Hagino M, Koizumi H, Otani H, Yano Y, Takada N (1994) A case report of *Diphyllobothriosis latum* we recently experienced, and the epidemiology of the same disease at the basin of the river Kugury. Clin Parasitol 5:186–187 (in Japanese)

Harada T, Sato N, Hagiwara T, Nozawa A, Takano Y, Takakuwa M (1992) Two cases of *Diphyllobothrium latum*. J Jpn Assoc Rural Med 41:46 (in Japanese)

Hokama S, Toda T, Kusano N, Nakamura H, Nakasone I, Nagamine T, Urasaki H, Chinen S, Kinjoh N, Sakiyama K, Yohena K, Taira S, Kyan T, Ohshiro M (1996) Recent features of parasites detected from clinical specimens. Jpn J Clin Pathol 44:379–383 (in Japanese with English abstract)

Hoshino H, Wada J, Okamoto K, Harasawa J, Nakayama S, Saito N, Konsei T, Yamazaki M, Uchida R, Shiohara T (1996) Two recent cases of *Diphyllobothrium latum*. Proc Jpn Soc Intern 440th Meet Kanto area. p 135 (in Japanese)

Ito R, Kodama H, Horie T, Ishii N, Chiba M, Masamune K (1991) Four cases of causative on *Diphyllobothrium latum*. Clin Parasitol 2:96–98 (in Japanese)

Iwata Y, Uehara M, Iwata M, Karino S, Suzuki M, Ichihara A, Kamegai T (1993) A case of *Diphyllobothrium nihonkaiense* which ejected perfectly by treatment before large intestine endoscopy. Clin Parasitol 4:97–98 (in Japanese)

Kihara T, Kobayashi R, Kosaka K (1973) Studies on large tapeworm. Part 2. The epidemiological and clinical studies of the broad tapeworm (*Diphyllobothrium latum*). Jpn J Gastroenterol 70:189–195 (in Japanese with English abstract)

Maejima J, Yazaki S, Fukumoto S (1991) Comparative studies on egg-sizes and forms of various *Diphyllobothrium* species from man in Japan. Jpn J Parasitol 40:170–176 (in Japanese with English abstract)

Maejima J, Yazaki S, Fukumoto S (1991) Egg size of *Diphyllobothrium nihonkaiense*. Jpn J Parasitol 40(suppl):67 (in Japanese)

Matsuura T, Bylund G, Sugane K (1992) Comparison of restriction fragment length polymorphisms of ribosomal DNA between *Diphyllobothrium nihonkaiense* and *D. latum*. J Helminthol 66:261–266

Mori T, Shimada M, Irino H (1991) Study on histological observation of *Diphyllobothrium latum* (in Japanese). Igakukensa (Jpn J Med Tech; JMT) 4:879–883

Nakayoshi A, Kuniyoshi T, Uechi H, Ooshiro J, Shikiya T, Aragaki T, Sakugawa H, Arakawa T, Kaneshiro F, Saito A (1990) Four cases of *Diphyllobothrium* which ejected by gastrografin. Clin Parasitol 1:116–118 (in Japanese)

Nishikawa S, Hosomi M, Kosaka T, Tsujiai T, Furukawa K, Sakagami T, Tanida H, Shitamoma T (1992) Three cases of causative on *Diphyllobothrium latum*. Clin Parasitol 3:138–139 (in Japanese)

Nishiyama T, Amano H, Kimoto M, Araki T, Ishizaka S (1995) A case of infection with four *Diphyllobothrium nihonkaiense* worms treated with praziquantel. Clin Parasitol 6:69–72 (in Japanese)

Ohnishi K, Murata M (1994) Praziquantel for the treatment of *Diphyllobothrium nihonkaiense* infections in humans. Trans R Soc Trop Med Hyg 88:580

Ozaki M, Nakajima Y, Tomii S, Yoshida M, Kurihara K, Watanabe S, Abe T, Utsunomiya K, Takahashi S, Saito M, Aoyanagi T (1990) An examinatioin of *Diphyllobothrium latum* in medical treatment by infusing of gastrografin. Clin Parasitol 1:119–121 (in Japanese)

Sugawara K, Hoshihara Y, Yamamoto T, Okuda C, Kimura T, Iguchi D, Tanaka T, Yamamoto N, Hashimoto M (1996) A case of *Diphyllobothrium latum* infection unexpectedly found during colonoscopy. Prog Dig Endosc 49:208–209 (in Japanese with English abstract)

Sugi K, Saito N, Nakagawa H, Sugimori K, Hirata I,Oshiba S (1993) An examination of *Diphyllobothrium latum* experienced at Osaka Medical University. Clin Parasitol 4:117–123 (in Japanese)

Tada M, Iso A, Otsuka H, Shimizu S, Aoki Y, Okamura M (1990) Parasitology of *Diphyllobothrium latum* in small intestine. Clin Parasitol 1:110–113 (in Japanese)

Takayama N (1996) Four cases of *Diphyllobothrium nihonkaiense* infection in a child (in Japanese). Tokyo Metropolitan Government Public Health Acadany Journal 70:338–339 (in Japanese)

Taya T, Yazaki Y, Kitagawa T, Ishikawa Y, Yoshida K, Sekiya C, Namiki M (1990) Medical treatment on many numbers of parasitic cases of *Diphyllobothrium latum*. Clin Parasitol 1:122–123 (in Japanese)

Yamaguchi T, Kamoshida S, Yokoda K, Shimizu T, Morita T, Okada Y, Matsuda M, Kanou M, Iwasaki A, Arakawa T (1994) Two cases of broad tapeworm infection. Clin Parasitol 5:184–185 (in Japanese)

Yamane Y, Kamo H, Bylund G, Wikgren Bo-Jungar P (1986) *Diphyllobothrium nihonkaiense* sp. nov. (cestoda: *Diphyllobothriidae*) revised indentification of Japanese broad tapeworm. Shimane J Med Sci 10:29–48

Yamane Y, Yoneyama T, Hokujo N, Fukushima T, Enho T, Oshita M, Imaoka T (1993) 12 cases of *Diphyllobothrium nihonkaiense* in Shimane and its epidemiological examination. Clin Parasitol 4:114–116 (in Japanese)

Yanagisawa R, Kawakami T, Nakamura K, Kojima H, Suzuki H, Suzuki A, Uchida A, Murata Y, Tamai Y (1996) Glycosphingolipid's structure of glycochaine from *Diphyllobothrium nihonkaiense*. Jpn J Pathol 68:602 (in Japanese)

Yazaki Y, Namiki M (1983) The effect of paromomycin sulfate on *Diphyllobothrium latum*. Jpn J Antibiot 36:613–614 (in Japanese with English abstract)

Parasitology and International Health

Isao Tada

Summary. A recent trend in the presentations at the annual meetings of the Japanese Society of Parasitology during these past 30 years has been a gradual and steady increase in papers concerning overseas research activities, particularly after the mid-1970s. Since several years ago, this rate has attained 10% and more of the total presentations. This tendency can be attributed to fact that many Japanese parasitologists have looked for incentive in developing countries following the marked postwar reduction of domestic parasitic infections. It should be noted that in the field conditions of developing countries, various diagnostic methods have been developed, as shown in the table. Recently, emerging and reemerging parasitic diseases such as infection with *Plasmodium* are threatening mankind. From this view, cooperation and collaboration between parasitology and agencies of international health are considered enormously important for the control of diseases.

Key Words: Parasitology—International health—Diagnosis—Control—Developing country—Japanese Society of Parasitology—Trend—Presentation—Parasitic disease—Emerging/reemerging disease—ODA—Grant—Research

Introduction

One of the marked trends in parasitology in Japan during these past several decades is the commitment to overseas research activities, particularly within the framework of international health projects. For example, the presentations at the annual meetings of the Japanese Society

Department of Parasitology, Faculty of Medicine, Kyushu University, 3-1-1 Maidashi, Higashi-ku, Fukuoka 812-8582, Japan

of Parasitology during these 30 years have shown a gradual and steady increase in papers dealing with research activities abroad, especially after the mid-1970s. The average total of the presentations in an annual meeting is about 150, while the percentage of research in developing tropical countries has increased gradually from approximately 2% before 1970 to 6% between 1976 and 1990. However, in the past several years, this rate has been enhanced remarkably to more than 10% of the total presentations (14% in 1996). This tendency can be attributed to the fact that many Japanese parasitologists have looked for incentive and materials in developing tropical countries following the marked postwar reduction of domestic parasitic infections.

Overseas Research

Research abroad includes the following categories: (1) epidemiology of various parasitic infections, (2) biology of pathogenic parasites and their vector/intermediate host, (3) biology of parasite transmission, (4) diagnosis of parasitic infections, (5) study of the control of target parasitic infections, and (6) new records of parasites from humans and animals (including the description of new species). Many of these research activities were supported mainly by grants from the Ministry of Education and Official Development Assistance (ODA) projects by the aid agency JICA (Japan International Cooperation Agency). The importance of the latter agency is noticeable. In the latter category, however, international health collaboration is the major purpose, even when it includes applied investigations in the field. Therefore, the balance between research and technical collaboration and transfer has been an important concern for parasitologists in any project so far. However, it should be stressed that the main objective of parasitologists involved has been parasitology, but not the health issue itself. It may thus be said they chose tropical countries as alternatives to the domestic field where only a few parasites occur and the necessary tools and methodology were already established for many parasitic infections.

Research Within International Health Programs

In many universities in Japan, the shortage of research grants has been worrying researchers for a long time. In fiscal 1985, the total of research grants offered by the Ministry of Education to all university and college faculties was 42 billion yen, and the approval rate for new applications was 23.2%. In the year 1996, however, grants were increased to 101.8 billion yen and more than 30%, respectively. Considering the low basic budget for each department, these numbers are quite small on a per capita basis. Usually a department that includes four or five faculties in an ordinary medical school in any national university has been nurtured by an annual budget of about 2.5–3.5 million yen for about 30 years. To improve the quality of research facilities, it is concluded that the financial barrier has thus been tremendous. On the other hand, the Official Development Assistance (ODA) of Japan has been increasing on a year-by-year basis, and the amount of money spent in the international health program in recipient developing countries has also been great recently. An average research-type health collaboration project by the Japan International Cooperation Agency (JICA) has been spending about 250 million yen for 5 years. Even when expenditure for the infrastructure is subtracted from this amount, an individual project is able to invest a short-term but sufficient amount for research activities. In comparison with the research grant by the Ministry of Education (average, 5 million yen, mainly for travel expense) for an average overseas research project, there is a marked difference (Tada 1996).

Contribution to Diagnosis

In this context, it should be noted that privilege and merit are provided by a long-term stay in developing countries with favorable conditions (laboratory devices and reagents, transportation, counterparts, authorization, etc.) based on international health projects. However, at the same time, there are various disadvantages, such as the time-consuming effort required in technical transfer, which tend to diminish research activities, production of scientific papers with high impact factor, and contact with up-to-date scientific information in the same area. Despite the presence of such unfavorable conditions, parasitologists have been engaging in such research based on individual interests. Among those investigations, I give some examples of technical standardization and improvements in the diagnosis of parasitic infections. This type of research, as mentioned in the following list, has been promoted in these favorable environments within the framework of international health projects (Table 1):

1. Parasitological diagnosis: the skin-snipping method was standardized in endemic areas of onchocerciosis; acridine-orange staining method was developed for the rapid detection of *Plasmodium* in the blood, and

Table 1. Examples of diagnostic methods for parasitic infections improved in some international health collaborations

Diagnostic methods	Target parasites	Projects (country)
Skin snipping	*Onchocerca volvulus*	Onchocerciosis research (Guatemala) (Tada et al. 1979)
IHA	*Onchocerca volvulus*	Onchocerciosis Research (Guatemala) (Ikeda et al. 1978)
ELISA	*Onchocerca volvulus*	Onchocerciosis research (Guatemala/Nigeria) (Korenaga et al. 1983)
Rapid diagnosis by fluorescence micro-scopy	*Plasmodium* sp.	Malaria control (Solomon) (Kawamoto et al. 1991)
DNA diagnosis	*Plasmodium*	Malaria control (Solomon) (Wataya et al. 1993)
G-6-PD deficiency	*Plasmodium*	Malaria control (Solomon) (Matsuoka et al. 1986)
Urine examination	*Schistosoma haematobium*	Kenyan Medical Research Institute (Kenya) (Shimada et al. 1986)
Gelatin particle agglutination	*Trypanosoma cruzi*	Community Health (Paraguay)
PCR diagnosis	*Plasmodium*	Research of tropical diseases (Malaysia) (Noor Rain et al. 1996)
PCR diagnosis	*Entamoeba histolytica/ E. dispar*	LIKA (Brazil) (Tachibana et al. 1992)
Dipstick method	*Schistosoma haematobium*	Noguchi Project (Ghana) (Bosompem et al. 1996)
IFA	*Plasmodium*	Malaria control (Sudan) (Kano et al. 1993)

IHA, indirect hemagglutination assay; G-6-PD, glucose-6-phosphate dehydrogenase; PCR, polymerase chain reaction; IFA, indirect fluorescent assay.

improvement of the measurement method for egg output and hematuria was made in the urine examination for *Schistosoma haematobium* infection.

2. Immunodiagnosis: Various techniques of immunodiagnosis such as indirect hemagglutination, enzyme-linked immunosorbent assay (ELISA), avidin-biotin complex (ABC-) ELISA, immunodiffusion, gelatin particle agglutination, and monoclonal antibody-based dipstick assays

were standardized in onchocerciosis, Chagas disease, schistosomosis, malaria (diagnostic and epidemiological assessment), echinococcosis, etc. To obtain various antigens, natural and social conditions in the developing countries are favorable for the collection of various species of parasites.

3. Molecular biological diagnosis: polymerase chain reaction (PCR) was applied to the differentiation between *Entamoeba histolytica* and *E. dispar*. The plate hybridization method for the detection of *Plasmodium* in the blood was also realized.

4. Other: improvement of agar gel method to detect glucose-6-phosphate dehydrogenase (G-6-PD) deficiency, which is necessary in the administration of some antimalarial drugs.

The qualification of such techniques was clearly attained under such favorable conditions as a sufficient number of patients, biopsy/serum samples, parasite/antigens, and clinical needs.

To perform research work within the framework of international health projects on the ODA basis, a parasitologist has to conquer a variety of disadvantages as mentioned earlier. Some recommended solutions are (1) to utilize the Internet for communication and literature searching, (2) to find proper research targets under field conditions and with merits as mentioned here, and (3) to cement unity with appropriate counterparts as co-workers and adapt to foreign cultures. Recently, emerging and reemerging parasites such as *Plasmodium* are arousing much controversy as a threat to mankind. From this aspect, combination and collaboration between parasitology and international health is considerably important. This partnership is valuable not only for the standardization and improvement of diagnostic methodologies of parasitic infections, but also for the development of specialists in this field of science, parasitology.

References

Bosompem KM, et al (1996) Limited field evaluation of a rapid monoclonal antibody-based dipstick assay for urinary schistosomosis. Hybridoma 15:443–447

Ikeda T, et al (1978) The indirect hemagglutination test for onchocerciosis performed with blood collected on filter paper. J Parasitol 64:786–789

Korenaga M, et al (1983) Enzyme-linked immunosorbent assay (ELISA) in the detection of IgG antibodies in onchocerciosis using blood collected on filter paper. Jpn J Parasitol 32:347–355

Kano S, et al (1993) Antibody frequency distribution curve for risk assessment of a malaria epidemic in the Sudan. Jpn J Trop Med Hyg 21:207–211

Kawamoto F, et al (1991) Rapid diagnosis of malaria by fluorescence microscopy using an interference filter and a daylight-illuminated microscope. Jpn J Trop Med Hyg 19(suppl):64

Matsuoka H, et al (1986) Malaria and glucose-6-phosphate dehydrogenase deficiency in North Sumatra, Indonesia. Southeast Asian J Trop Med Public Health 17:530–536

Noor Rain A, et al (1996) Development of a new diagnostic method for *Plasmodium falciparum* infection using a reverse transcriptase-polymerase chain reaction. Am J Trop Med Hyg 54:162–163

Shimada M, et al (1986) Egg count in urine to determine the intensity of *Schistosoma haematobium* infection. Jpn J Trop Med Hyg 14:267–272

Tachibana H, et al (1992) Analysis of pathogenicity by restriction-endonuclease digestion of amplified genomic DNA of *Entamoeba histolytica* isolated in Pernambuco, Brazil. Parasitol Res 78:433–436

Tada I, et al (1979) Onchocerciosis in San Vicente Pacaya, Guatemala. Am J Trop Med Hyg 28:67–71

Tada I (1996) Parasitology and international health collaborations: advantage and disadvantage. Jpn J Parasitol 45:465–473

Wataya Y, et al (1993) DNA diagnosis of falciparum malaria using a double PCR technique: a field trial in the Solomon Islands. Mol Biochem Parasitol 58:165–168

Yamashita T, et al (1994) The gelatin particle indirect agglutination test, a means of simple and sensitive serodaiganosis of Chagas disease. Jpn J Trop Med Hyg 22:5–8

Pathology of Parasitic Zoonoses

HIDEYO ITAKURA and KAN TORIYAMA

Summary. Pathologists today have insufficient appreciation of the broad societal significance of parasitic diseases and their impact on the world. Responding to the need for a clear and consistent pathological approach, our presentation sets out characteristic histopathological features of parasitic diseases. Focused on common parasitic diseases such as leishmaniosis, amebosis, schistosomosis, opisthorchiosis, echinococcosis, cysticercosis, and trichinosis, this chapter makes abundant use of histopathological materials in our case library. The pathological changes that parasites induce in their hosts are caused by a variety of mechanisms. Many pathogenic parasitic infections are known as parasitic zoonoses. Parasitic diseases are distributed as endemic diseases in many parts of the world, especially in the tropics and subtropics.

Key Words: Histopathological features—Parasitic diseases—Leishmaniosis—Amebosis—Schistosomosis—Opisthorchiosis—Echinococcosis—Cysticercosis—Trichinosis—Parasitic zoonoses—Endemic diseases—Tropics—Subtropics—Wild animals—Vectors

Introduction

This symposium on the pathology of parasitic zoonoses incorporating the contributions of distinguished symposists was organized in response to the needs of the current period. Because of current social and economic trends, human populations have begun to grow and to move to other areas of the world. Parasitic worms infect humans in almost all regions of the world. It is often perceived that cultural food habits and local prac-

Department of Pathology, Institute of Tropical Medicine, Nagasaki University, 1-12-4 Sakamoto, Nagasaki 852-8523, Japan

tices contribute to the incidence of parasitic infections in man. Parasitic diseases have been becoming relatively frequent as the result of changes in lifestyle as well as an increased variety of personal food habits. Some parasitic diseases are resurgent in many countries. Parasitic diseases spread as people increasingly travel through or reside in areas of the world with poor sanitation. Parasitic diseases have recently become frequent in so-called economically advanced countries as practices of feeding domestic animals and importing animals for scientific experiments or importing foods from tropical and subtropical countries have become more common.

In Japan, economic success has brought about the improvement of environmental hygiene and medical facilities and practice as well as the increased awareness and promotion of public health. These changes have resulted in the eradication of most of the parasitic diseases in the country. However, parasitic diseases remain a major problem worldwide and may even be spreading as a result of the greenhouse effect. Moreover, parasitic disease is regaining importance because of importation as well as travel-related transmission resulting from Japan's increasing internationalization.

There is, however, a disturbing misconception inherent in the term "parasitology," for some parasitic diseases are not exotic on the domestic scene. Pathologists today have insufficient appreciation of the broad societal significance of parasitic diseases and their impact on the world. The immediate diagnosis and treatment of patients with incipient parasitic disease are essential. Nevertheless, the pathogenesis of most parasitic diseases remains to be elucidated and the histopathological diagnosis of the disease often meets with difficulty. Parasitic zoonoses, in other words, the parasitic diseases common between man and animals, are still important.

Responding to the need for a clear and consistent pathological approach, our presentation sets out characteristic histopathological features of parasitic diseases needed to facilitate a provisional or definitive diagnosis (Marcial-Rojas 1971; Hunter et al. 1976; Doerr and Seifert 1995; Orihel and Ash 1995).

Materials and Methods

Focused on common parasitic diseases, this presentation makes abundant use of histopathological materials in our case library, which have been collected from various parts of Africa, Southeast Asia, and Japan.

Among the study materials, biopsy and surgical specimens of parasitic diseases, with information about age, sex, ethnic group, and residence area in western Kenya, East Africa, that have been examined histopathologically for more than 20 years were included.

Results and Discussion

Visceral leishmaniosis (kala-azar) is a disseminated infection by the protozoan *Leishmania donovani*. Within phagocytic cells of the soft connective tissues, reticuloendothelial system, and blood of its mammalian host, *L. donovani* occurs as an intracytoplasmic round or ovoid body (L-D body). In hematoxylin-eosin preparations, L-D bodies usually can be clearly demonstrated in well-fixed tissues. It is necessary to differentiate L-D bodies from *Histoplasma capsulatum* or other yeastlike fungus cells, *Toxoplasma gondii*, and the leishmaniform bodies of *Trypanosoma cruzi*. Liver biopsy specimens of visceral leishmaniosis of an African male patient with hepatosplenomegaly and hyperglobulinemia showed histologically marked inflammatory exudate of plasma cells, lymphocytes, and macrophages mainly in portal areas of the hepatic lobules. L-D bodies were found in macrophages and in Kupffer's cells. L-D bodies were also observed in hepatocytes in some parts of the lobules. Characteristic intracellular organelles of the protozoa such as the nucleus, kinetoplast, and axoneme were found by electron microscopic examination. The protozoa was confirmed to be in a mastigote stage. Histopathological differential diagnosis of kala-azar from other chronic liver diseases such as chronic viral hepatitis is important (Yamashita et al. 1979).

Cutaneous leishmaniosis is mainly caused by *Leishmania tropica*. The lesion begins as papules or nodules which are associated with underlying bulging inflammatory cells in the dermis. The inflammatory cells consist of lymphocytes, monocytes, histiocytes, and plasma cells. *Leishmania* are found mostly within the cytoplasm of histiocytes. In the early stages of the disease, the lesion is histologically characterized by moderate proliferation of histiocytes containing numerous parasites (Figs. 1 and 2). Multiple lesions are not uncommon. The papules become moist and form a crust that falls away, leaving an ulcer.

Amebosis is caused by *Entamoeba histolytica* and shows a worldwide distribution. *E. histolytica* is primarily a parasite of the gastrointestinal tract. Infection begins when the parasite invades the mucosa of the colon (Fig. 3). All other localizations of amebae are either secondary to this particular lesion or represent extremely rare occurrences. In many cases

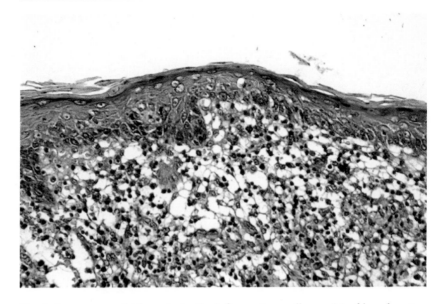

Fig. 1. In cutaneous leishmaniosis, the inflammatory cells consist of lymphocytes, monocytes, histiocytes, and plasma cells

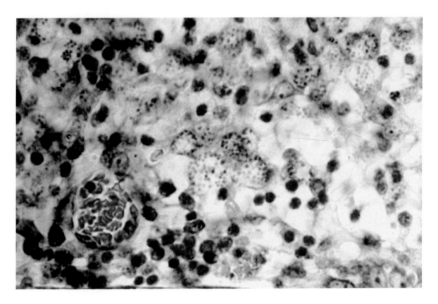

Fig. 2. In cutaneous leishmaniosis, the diffuse infiltrate of histiocytes contains numerous intracytoplasmic parasites

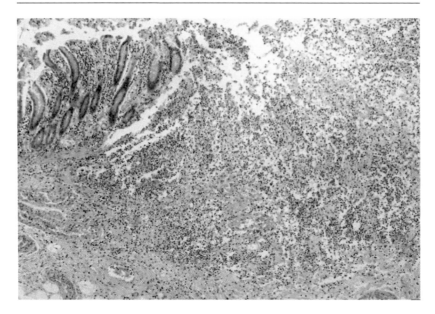

Fig. 3. In amebosis, an ulcer in the colon shows a superficial type of necrosis and an overhanging edge of preserved mucosa

of amebosis in adults, abscess formations of the liver are observed. Although the most common organ of metastatic infection is the liver, other organs such as the lungs, brain, genital organs, and skin may be involved. One of the peculiar aspects of amebosis is the scanty inflammation of infected foci.

Schistosomosis haematobia, caused by *Schistosoma haematobium*, is widely distributed all over Africa. The urinary bladder is the organ affected earliest and most severely and constantly. Cystitis usually manifests itself in young persons between the ages of 10 and 30 years. The ova, deposited mostly in the submucosa, elicit a reaction of the surrouding tissues leading to the formation of granulomas (Fig. 4). Although the general consensus of opinion is that cancer of the bladder is related to urinary schistosomosis, the exact relationship still remains obscure, and much work is needed to clarify the role of the disease in the pathogenesis of bladder cancer (Fig. 5).

Opisthorchiosis, caused by species of *Opisthorchis* that live in the bile ducts of humans and animals, may be seen in Asia and other areas (Fig. 6). Echinococcosis or hydatidosis is one of the most important zoonoses

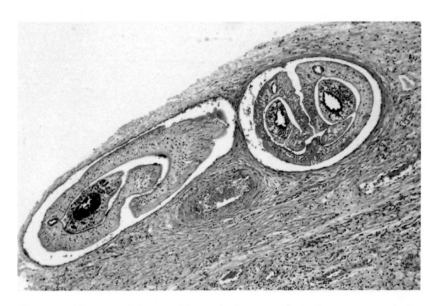

Fig. 4. In schistosomosis haematobia, a pair of connected parasites are present in the testicular tissue of a young Kenyan boy

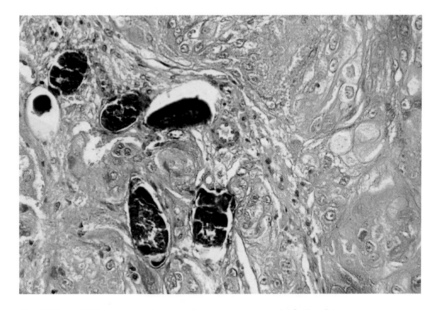

Fig. 5. In schistosomosis haematobia, numerous calcified schistosome eggs are evident in the mucosa of the urinary bladder. Although the exact relationship still remains obscure, carcinoma of the bladder may be related to urinary schistosomosis. Note that the tumor is not transitional cell carcinoma but squamous cell carcinoma

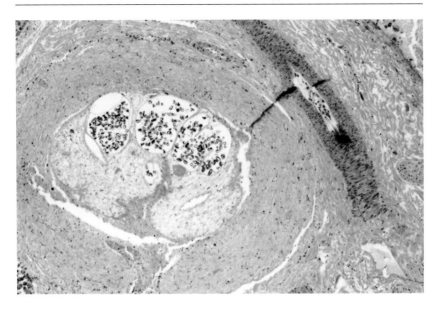

Fig. 6. Opisthorchiosis, showing blocking of the bile ducts by parasites

in many parts of the world. Unilocular hydatid disease caused by *Echinococcus granulosus* is prevalent in Africa and other tropical areas. The main lesion is formation of cysts as large as 20 cm in diameter (Fig. 7). The lesions are most commonly found in the liver, omentum, mesentery, and abdominal wall. The large cyst formation of this disease causes mechanical and functional disturbances of the affected organs.

Cysticercosis is found in all parts of the world where *Taenia solium* is present. Human cysticercosis occurs when humans accidentally become the intermediate host of *T. solium*. The type of lesions, observed in any part of the body, that may harbor cysticerci depends on the time that has elapsed following infection. The central nervous system, eyes, and skin constitute a relatively common localization for the parasites. Microscopic lesions in the central nervous system vary according to the viability of the parasite. When the parasite is viable, almost no inflammatory reaction is seen. On the other hand, when the parasite is dead, several features of the inflammatory reaction are present.

The ingestion of meat that contains viable cysts of *Trichinella spiralis* is followed by a disease of variable intensity and duration in humans and other mammals known as trichinosis, trichinelliasis, trichinellosis, or

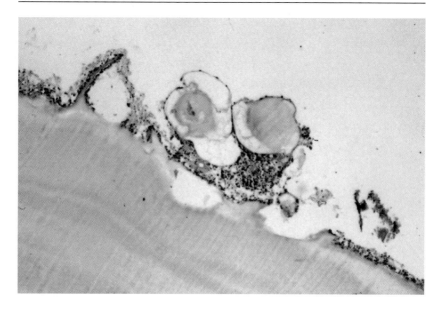

Fig. 7. Echinococcosis: a unilocular hydatid cyst

trichiniasis. The coiled larva encysting in human muscle fibers is seen microscopically. The muscle fibers subsequently undergo degeneration or necrosis. Edema, hyperemia, and an interstitial infiltrate that contains many histiocytes, leukocytes, and eosinophils are observed (Fig. 8).

According to our geopathological study of parasitic zoonoses in western Kenya, East Africa, dermal leishmaniosis is most common, followed by unilocular echinococcosis, schistosomosis haematobia, amebic dysentery, cystisercosis, and dracunculiosis (dracontosis, dracunculosis) (Toriyama et al. 1997). Most cases of leishmaniosis in our study were cutaneous leishmaniosis, in which ulcer formations were seen in the face and extremities. Children were more commonly affected than adults. Echinococcosis was prevalent in dry areas of northwestern Kenya and in the lake basin of Lake Victoria. Almost all cases of schistosomosis examined in western Kenya were schistosomosis haematobia. The disease is also very common in the surrounding areas of Lake Victoria. The majority of patients with this disease were young people. The main viscera affected were the urinary bladder, vagina, and rectum. A case of coenurosis examined by us showed characteristic anatomical features of the parasites (Fig. 9). These results were obtained only from the cases in

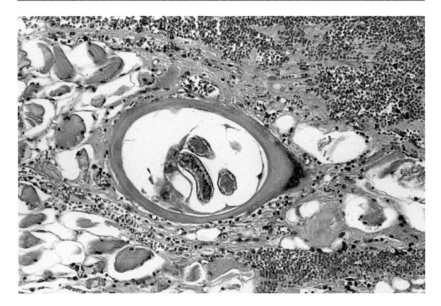

Fig. 8. In trichinosis, coiled larva encysting in human muscle fibers

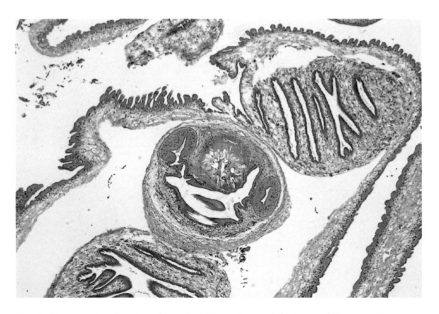

Fig. 9. Coenurosis, showing characteristic anatomical features of the parasites

which histological examinations were available. Many of the patients who suffered from parasitic diseases are living in the desert or semidesert areas in tropical Africa.

The pathological changes that parasites induce in their hosts are the effects of a variety of mechanisms. The pathological effects of parasites may be interference with absorption of food, competition for nutrients, mechanical disturbance such as obstruction and space-occupying lesions, chemical injury by toxic metabolites, and immunological reactions caused by antigens of the metabolites.

Many pathogenic parasitic infections are known as parasitic zoonoses. Parasitic diseases are distributed as endemic diseases in many parts of the world, especially in the tropics and subtropics. Opportunities for contact with contaminated water of rivers or lakes, drinking water, the meat of domestic or wild animals, and vectors should be avoided when one travels or lives in such areas.

References

Doerr HW, Seifert G (1995) Tropical pathology. Spezielle pathologische Anatomie. Springer, Berlin Heidelberg New York

Hunter GW III, Swartzwelder JC, Clyde DF (1976) Tropical medicine. Saunders, Philadelphia

Marcial-Rojas RA (1971) Pathology of protozoal and helminthic diseases. Williams and Wilkins, Baltimore

Orihel TC, Ash LR (1995) Parasites in human tissues. American Society of Clinical Pathologists, Chicago

Toriyama K, Kusuda M, Itakura H (1997) Epidemiology and geopathology of parasitic zoonoses in western Kenya (in Japanese). 34th Conf Jpn Assoc African Stud Abstr 47

Yamashita H, Senba M, Itakura H (1979) Histopathology of liver biopsy of kala-azar. Trop Med 23(3):127–130

The Taxonomic Study of Diphyllobothriid Cestodes with Special Reference to *Diphyllobothrium nihonkaiense* in Japan

Yosuke Yamane, Kuninori Shiwaku, Tetsuhito Fukushima, Akio Isobe, Gao Tong Qiang, and Toshimi Yoneyama

Summary. The epidemiological features of diphyllobothriosis nihonkaiense are described. The case incidence showed peaks in the 1920s, 1970s, and 1980s. The geographic distribution covers all Japan. The main subjective symptoms are evacuation (83%), diarrhea or loose bowels (14%), and abdominal pain (13%). The taxonomic features of *Diphyllobothrium nihonkaiense* are described according to the following points: the shape and size of the scolex, bothrium development, neck length, segment form and size, segmental surface structure, internal structure, form and size of egg, pattern of egg-surface pits, growth condition of coracidia, form and size of hooks of the hexacanth embryo, form and size of the plerocercoid, bothrial slit, and tail excavation, and transverse furrows of the body surface. As for the internal structure of the plerocercoid, microtriches, the subtegumental and longitudinal muscle layer, parenchymal longitudinal muscle layer, subtegumental cell layer, and distribution of frontal gland showed as marked features. The physiological, biochemical, and molecular phylogenic features have been applied to species identification. We have tried to analyze the trace element content, amino acid content, isozyme pattern, immunological specificity, and DNA sequences. The natural focus of *D. nihonkaiense* is not yet defined, but the intermediate host, the masu salmon, *Oncorhynchus masou*, spawns all around the Sea of Okhotsk and the Sea of Japan.

Key Words: Cestode—Clinical parasitology—Diphyllobothriid cestode—*Diphyllobothrium nihonkaiense*—Ecology—Epidemiology—Fish parasite—Japan Sea—Masu salmon—Natural focus—Paleoparasitology—Prevention—Tapeworm—Taxonomy—Therapy

Department of Environmental Medicine, Shimane Medical University, 89 Enya, Izumo, Shimane 693-8501, Japan

Introduction

Human diphyllobothriosis is known to be widely distributed in the world, but there are considerable lacunae or inaccuracies in our knowledge as to the specific identity, distribution, epidemiology, biology, clinical features, and ecology of diphyllobothriid cestodes.

Human diphyllobothriosis cases have recently increased in Japan, reflecting the change of people's dietary habits. More and more Japanese people now travel or live abroad with chances to try rare foods, while thanks to the highly developed distribution system people in Japan can now taste various foreign and domestic fresh foods. Opportunities to enjoy outdoor life have also increased.

This report analyzes cases of diphyllobothriosis with special reference to *Diphyllobothrium nihonkaiense* as reported in Japan from historical, epidemiological, taxonomic, and ecological aspects.

History

The earliest references in Japanese medical literature to diphyllobothriid cestode infection were made in the old Japanese books of traditional medicine, such as Tsumura Soan's *Tankai* (1795), and in *Shinsen-Yamainosoushi* (1850: author unknown) (Fig. 1). In these books it is

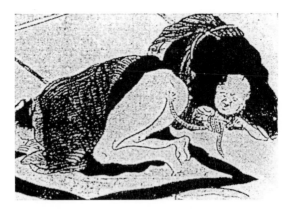

Fig. 1. The oldest description of diphyllobothriid cestode infection in Japan appeared in the traditional medical book *Shinsen-Yamainosoushi*, published in the eighteenth century

described as a long white worm that causes abdominal pain, and which is discharged from the anus at the time of evacuation, at which time it is suggested not to pull the worm out hastily because the worm is easy to break off. The infection was described as being acquired from eating raw salmon. As salmon was a popular dish in the Edo period, diphyllobothriid cestode infection, probably caused by *Diphyllobothrium nihonkaiense*, might have been also well known then.

Going back to ancient times, our paleoparasitological investigation on soil taken from the ruins of toilets in the ancient city of Fujiwara-kyo (674–710 A.D.) disclosed the existence of eggs of *Ascaris lumbricoides* (fertilized and unfertilized eggs), *Trichuris trichiura*, *Diphyllobothrium nihonkaiense*, *Metagonimus yokogawai*, and *Clonorchis sinensis*. So, it became clear that the Japanese had already begun to eat raw masu salmon (*Oncorhynchus masou*) in the seventh century and were infected with *Diphyllobothrium nihonkaiense*.

In Japan, *Diphyllobothrium nihonkaiense* was considered to be the same species as *Diphyllobothrium latum* for a long time. Here, I trace briefly the research history of the worm.

Iijima (1889) found that the infectious source of *Diphyllobothrium latum* in Japan was masu salmon, *Oncorhynchus masou*. Since Eguchi (1926) revealed the whole life cycle of *Diphyllobothrium latum*, human cases have been continuously reported, and have increased especially from the 1970s to the present. However, Kamo (1978) proposed reconsideration of the taxonomic status of *Diphyllobothrium latum* in Japan, with special reference to species-specific characters, on the basis of the concise observations of *Diphyllobothrium latum* (Linnaeus, 1758) and in light of the most advanced knowledge acquired by investigators in the Baltic region. Yamane et al. (1986) determined the taxonomic differences between *Diphyllobothrium latum* in Finland and in Japan with the cooperation of Åbo Akademi of Finland, and named *D. latum* in Japan as *Diphyllobothrium nihonkaiense* sp. nov. (Cestoda: Diphyllobothriidae).

Epidemiology

The epidemiology of diphyllobothriosis in Japan is characterized by three features. First, diphyllobothriosis is geographically distributed throughout Japan. Second, human cases have been increasing recently as a result of the gourmet tastes of contemporary Japanese. Third, 11 species have been reported as human diphyllobothriid cestodes in Japan since 1882 (Table 1). The common species reported were *D. nihonkaiense, Diplogonoporus grandis,* and *Spirometra erinacei* (plerocercoid). The numbers of cases caused by the main species are *D. nihonkaiense* (with so-called *D. latum*), 1617 (87.2%); *D. yonagoense,* 17 (0.9%); and *Diplogonoporus grandis,* 198 (10.7%).

The incidence of diphyllobothriosis has changed in the past 90 years. Prominent peaks were observed in the 1920s, the 1970s, and the 1980s (Fig. 2). Endemic infection was observed as the peak in the 1920s. For the second peak, the background may be the gourmet dietary tendency associated with the development of the transportation system for fresh masu salmon. As for incidence by sex and age, the highest incidence is in the thirties and forties, and incidence is greater in men (67.0%) than in women (22.6%).

The distribution of *D. nihonkaiense* infections includes all Japan. Prefectures with many infective cases and the numbers and percentages of cases are as follow: Gifu, 587 (36.6%); Kyoto, 130 (8.1%), Ishikawa, 96 (6.0%); Akita, 89 (5.6%); Aomori, 78 (4.9%); Tokyo, 78 (4.9%); Hokkaido, 62; Nagano, 60; Chiba, 45; and Toyama, 33. Niigata, Saitama, Osaka, Okayama, Okinawa, Nara, and Hiroshima also had some cases. More cases have occurred in the northern and middle parts of Japan than in other parts. Recently, however, the differences in geographic distribution between areas have become less conspicuous because of the development of a transportation system for fresh masu salmon.

Table 1. Human diphyllobothriosis reported in Japan (1882–1995)

Species	Male	Female	Unknown	Total
Diphyllobothrium latum	1043	355	162	1560
Diphyllobothrium nihonkaiense	41	11	5	57
Diphyllobothrium yonagoense	16	0	1	17
Diphyllobothrium pacificum	6	0	0	6
Diphyllobothrium cameroni	1	0	0	1
Diphyllobothrium hians	1	0	0	1
Diphyllobothrium scoticum	1	0	0	1
Diphyllobothrium orcini	1	0	0	1
Spirometra erinacei (adult)	10	0	2	12
Diplogonoporus grandis	161	23	14	198
Diplogonoporus fukuokaensis	0	1	0	1

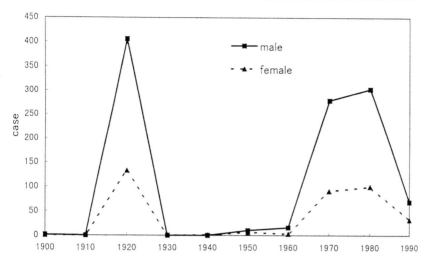

Fig. 2. Incidence of *Diphyllobothrium nihonkaiense* infection (1882–1995). *Squares,* males; *triangles,* females

Patients were distributed widely from infants to the elderly. The main occupations of patients are as follow: agriculture, 295 (34.3%); commerce, 155 (18.0%), schoolchildren and students, 70 (8.1%); and company employees, 69 (8.0%); public service, fisheries housewives, cooks, and teachers followed. As to the length of worms, 37.9% were less than 4 m, 22.8% were 4–6 m, 10.5% were 6–8 m, and 8.2% were longer than 8 m; the longest worm was 11.3 m.

The most frequent symptom of diphyllobothriosis nihonkaiense is the spontaneous evacuation of the strobila (62.1%), and after this, eggs in the feces (11.6%), diarrhea (8.2%), abdominal pain (5.1%), unusual abdominal sensations (2.9%), eosinophilia (2.6%), general fatigue (1.9%), followed by nausea and vomiting, dizziness, loss of weight, abdominal distension, and poor appetite. There was no difference in the symptoms between men and women (Fig. 3).

For therapy, paromomycin sulfate (49.1%), bithionol (24.4%), nicrosamide (5.7%), Gastrografin (5.1%), atebrin (4.5%), the Damaso de Rivas method (3.3%), and praziquantel (2.2%). Using these anthelmintics, the success rate was 81% with praziquantel, 57% with kamala, 54% with bithionol, 47% with the Damaso de Rivas method, and

case

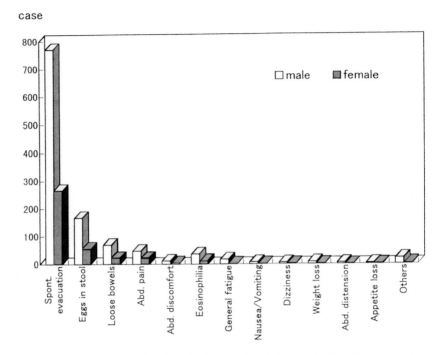

Fig. 3. *Chief complaints of Diphyllobothrium nihonkaiense* infection. *Spont.*, spontaneous; *abd.*, abdominal; *white*, males; *black*, females

28% in paromomycin sulfate. Of the patients, 88.7% were infected with a single worm, 5.3% had 2 worms, 2.4% had 3, and 1.6% had 4 worms; there was one case each with 5, 8, 13, 14, 32, and 43 worms. Clinical symptoms and laboratory data of diphyllobothriosis were obtained through experimental autoinfection. After swallowing 6 plerocercoids and keeping them within for 11 months, the patient showed general fatigue, abdominal pain, fever, diarrhea, and increase of eosinophil leucocytes to 21%.

We can summarize the epidemiological features of diphyllobothriosis nihonkaiense in Japan with these four points:

1. The case incidence showed peaks in the 1920s, 1970s, and 1980s. The highest incidence was in men in their thirties, and the ratio of male to female was 3:1.
2. The geographic distribution covered all Japan, and the infection occurred in children, students, and office workers.

3. The largest number of worms infecting one patient was 43. The main subjective symptoms were evacuation (83%), diarrhea or loose bowels (14%), and abdominal pain (13%).
4. For treatment, Gastrografin, paraziquantel, and bithionol were the most effective methods to preserve the scoleces.

Taxonomy

The establishment of systematic taxonomic criteria is important. The taxonomic features of diphyllobothriid cestodes have been obscured by the lack of reliable criteria, because *Dipyllobothrium* species are composed of soft tissues. Because it is very easy to alter the cestode by the anthelmintic drugs or fixation conditions used, it is very difficult to classify adult worms by morphological features alone. Therefore, we need to unify the identification method and taxonomic indices.

The taxonomic study of *Diphyllobothrium* has proceeded in Japan with the support of the fields of molecular biology, morphology, physiology, biochemistry, immunology, clinical medicine, epidemiology, and ecology, pursuing as comprehensively as possible the characteristics and character concordance of the species. Being conscious of the "species as the discontinuity between each group of individuals," parasitologists generally paid attention to morphological features (general external morphology, specific structures, internal morphology, and genetic and cellular characteristics), physiological features (metabolic, serological, biochemical, and secretory characteristics), ecological features (life history or life cycle, natural focus, seasonal variance, host–parasite relationship, and effects on the host), and geographic features (general distribution and geographic isolation of the species).

The body surface of *Diphyllobothrium*, lacking a cuticle, is liable to contraction and transformation if fixation is done in an unrelaxed state. Fixation must be carried out with sufficient relaxation of the body of the worm. Practically, the recommended method of fixation is as follows. First, cut off some segments filled with eggs from the strobila, which is previously washed with water. Put the separated segments in physiological saline to incubate the eggs and preserve them in a refrigerator at 4°C. Second, for biochemical and molecular biological analyses, cut off several segments and freeze them immediately. Third, for observation by electron microscopy, separate some other segments, cut them up into 1-mm^3 blocks, and fix them in 2.5% glutaraldehyde and 1% osmium tetroxide solution. Fourth, place the rest of the worm body in tap water containing chloroform (a few drops of chloroform for each 500 ml tap water), and preserve it in a refrigerator for several hours so that the worm will be relaxed and die. Fix some of the mature segments in 70% alcohol and the rest in 5% formalin. For the fixation of the plerocercoid, the Scandinavian method using 4% formol-saline (a mixture of formalin and physiological salt solution) is recommended.

Diphyllobothrium is inclined to show morphological characteristics more distinctly in the ploroceercoid stage than in the adult stage. Therefore, morphological and morphometric observations, especially scanning electron microscopic observations, are useful as taxonomic indices. Also, the possibility of applying progressive techniques of biochemistry, immunology, and molecular biology to parasite taxonomy is being investigated today.

As the taxonomic points of the strobila, the following information is useful: the shape and size of the scolex, bothrium development, neck length, segment form and size, segmental surface structure (furrows, genital papillae, situation of the genital pore and uterine pore of a segment), internal structure (microtriches, size and form of seminal vesicle and cirrus sac, location of cirrus sac, angle between the axis of the seminal vesicle and cirrus sac, uterine loop, horn formation of ovary, distribution of testes), form and size of egg, pattern of pits on the egg surface, growth condition of coracidia, hook form, and size of the hexacanth embryo.

In the diphyllobothriid cestode, the plerocercoid stage shows the most remarkable difference among species. The form and size of the plerocercoid, bothrial slit and tail excavation, and transverse furrows of body surface are helpful for identification. As for the internal structure of the plerocercoid, the microtriches, subtegumental and longitudinal muscle layer, parenchymal longitudinal muscle layer, subtegumental cell layer, and distribution of frontal gland are important as various morphological features. To distinguish these from species of marine origin, the pit pattern of the egg surface and the hatching conditions of eggs are also important indices.

Physiological, biochemical, and molecular phylogenic features have been applied recently to species identification. We have tried to analyze the prepatent period, growth and hatching of embryos in incubated eggs, shedding phenomenon of the plerocercoid, soluble protein profile, isozyme pattern, immunoelectrophoresis, trace element content, amino acid content, composition of lipids and fatty acids, isozyme pattern, im-munological specificity, and DNA sequences.

As for the relationship between host and parasite, the biological para-sitic dynamics of *Diphyllobothrium* after its infection have been revealed gradually. For instance, differences among species have been observed in the frequency of shedding phenomenon, that is, the active separation of the head part of the plerocercoid from the worm body, which happens soon after infection.

Profile of *Diphyllobothrium nihonkaiense*

An adult worm was experimentally reared in a golden hamster. The mean strobilar length was 693 mm, with about 633 segments. The maximum width, attained in gravid segments, was 6.9 mm. All the strobilae were attenuated with segmental margins indented. The mean width and length of gravid segments were 6.8 mm and 1.9 mm, respectively. The number of segments from the first segment to the primordium was 119, and the number of segments from the first segment to the mature proglottid was 444.

In each segment the width is greater than the length, and the length increases as the segment becomes closer to the end of strobila. The length to width ratio of immature segments is about 1:7 and that of gravid segments 1:3.5.

The scolex is mostly 2.6 mm long, 1.4 mm wide, and nearly spatulate in shape. There are numerous pits at the top of the scolex. The bothria is well developed, deep, and as long as the full length of the scolex. The neck is well developed, mostly 15.6 mm long and 1.22 mm wide.

The genital pore is situated ventrally on the midline at 260–340 µm posterior from the anterior margin of the segment, which is 1.9–2.1 mm in length. The uterine pore opens at 200–350 µm posterior from the genital pore.

The cirrus sac is oval and large, 420–480 µm in length by 390–400 µm in diameter, opening obliquely into the genital atrium. The seminal vesicle is also large and elliptical, 250 µm in length by 100 µm in diameter. It has a thick wall and is connected to the back of the cirrus sac making a sharp angle. The spherical testes, which are bulbs 35–45 µm in diameter, are arranged in a single layer in the medullary parenchyma, and are covered with a transverse muscle layer 5–10 µm in thickness. The testes are not distributed astride the boundary of segments.

The uterine loops, usually 6–7 loops, extend laterad, with peripheral loops opening into the uterine pore, not extending beyond the anterior margin of the genital atrium. The ovary is renal shaped, situated in the posterior margin of the segment, having neither anterior nor posterior horns.

Eggs in the uterine loops of strobilae reared in golden hamsters are ellipsoidal with an operculum, measuring 55.2 ± 1.3 μm in length by 38.2 ± 1.6 μm in diameter on average, the length/width ratio being 1.45 ± 0.06. Eggshells exhibit shallow pits distributed sparsely on the smooth surface.

The embryonal hooks are relatively short. The lengths of the first, second, and third hooks are 11.06 μm, 12.20 μm, and 12.35 μm, respectively. The ratio of blade length to total length of the hook is relatively large, 39.6% in the first hook, 36.2% in the second, and 37.4% in the third. The curvature of the second and third hook blades is deep and prominent, and the transitional slope from the blades to the guards is gentle. The hook guards are cylindrical and prominent, and project at right angles (90°) from the handle (Yamane et al. 1989).

Plerocercoids collected from masu salmon, and fixed in 4% formol-saline, are yellowish white and cylindrical. On average they are 8.2 mm long × 1.1 mm wide × 0.7 mm high. The body tapers slowly toward the tail, somewhat flattened dorsoventrally. The width is maximum at the middle of the body. The scolex is evaginated with dorsal and ventral median grooves like lips. The tail is concave concentrically. The bothrium extends dorsoventrally. The tegument is covered with regular transverse wrinkles that are 240–400 μm wide. Microtriches, 3.3 μm long, cover the tegumental surface. The tegument is 14.6 μm thick, and the subtegumental longitudinal muscle layer is 9.2 μm thick on average. The average number of muscle bundles within a 50-μm space is 31.6.

There are well-developed parenchymal longitudinal muscles, 85.7 μm thick. The muscle bundles are arranged densely, 119 within a 50-μm space. The subtegumental cell layer is extremely well developed, 36.8 μm thick. Parenchymal cells are also densely arranged, 34 in a 50-μm area. The frontal glands are distributed locally and concentrated in the top region, occupying 6.4% of the whole body.

As for the early developmental pattern in the golden hamster, *D. nihonkaiense* showed 67% shedding in 3 and 8 h after infection and 100% in 24 h. The shedding occurs at an early point, and the recovery rate of the worm was high, 100% in *D. nihonkaiense*, compared with the rate of 48.8% in *D. latum*.

The trace elements content (μg/g dry wt) in the strobilae are Ca, 5880; Na, 1480; Mg, 680; Cu, 303; Fe, 240; Mn, 35; and Cd, 9.7. The characteristics seemed to be an abundance of Cu, Zn, and Fe and a trace of Cd. The antigenic structures were examined by immunoelectrophoresis. From the results of cross-reactions by the absorption procedure with heterologous antigen, the characteristic bands for *D. nihonkaiense* proved to be 14, in contrast with 21 for *D. latum*. In the soluble protein profiles and isozyme patterns, *D. nihonkaiense* showed species-specific patterns in the soluble protein profiles and zymograms of two enzymes, esterase 1 and esterase D, and acid phospatase. Enzyme polymorphism was observed in the zymograms of malic enzyme and β-*N*-acetyl-glucosaminidase (Fukumoto et al. 1987, 1988).

In the analysis of fatty acid composition, *D. nihonkaiense* showed a high content of linoleic, eichosadienoic, arachidonic, eicosapentaenoic, dochosabutanoic, and dochosahexaenoic acid, and a low content of palmitic, stearic, and oleic, as compared with *D. latum* in Finland.

Amino acid composition has recently been used as a taxonomic indicator. In the case of *D. nihonkaiense*, serine, glycine, valine, isoleucine, tyrosine, and arginine showed a high content.

Ecology

Ecological features are also important in geographic distribution. The species of diphyllobothriid cestodes depend on the fish species of the second intermediate host, and distribution of cestodes is restricted by the natural foci of the fish (Groot and Margolis 1991). The main infectious sources of diphyllobothriosis nihonkaiense are the masu salmon, *Onchorhynchus masou*, and pink salmon (humpback), *Onchorhynchus gorbusha* (Machidori 1981). However, many kinds of salmonid fish are imported now, so we have to be more careful in identifying the species of diphyllobothriid cestodes.

There are three main natural foci of diphyllobothriid cestodes in the world: North Europe, Canada and North America, and the Far East. In the North European focus based in lakes, burbot, pike, ruff, Atlantic salmon, lake trout, grayling, and eel were reported as the second intermediate host of *D. latum*. In the Canada and North American focus, barred pike, American burbot, blue pike (wall-eyed), sand pike, sockeye salmon, masu salmon, and pink salmon were the second intermediate host of *D. latum* and *D. nihonkaiense*. In the Far Eastern focus, masu salmon and pink

salmon are known as the second intermediate host of *D. nihonkaiense*.
In the case of *D. nihonkaiense*, the intermediate host, masu salmon,
Oncorhynchus masou, spawn all around the Sea of Okhotsk, Kamchatka
Peninsula, and Sea of Japan and spawn up the rivers in Russia, Korea, and
Japan (Fig. 4).

To clarify the natural foci of *D. nihonkaiense*, we need to develop
international cooperation. Through a cooperative study with a Korean

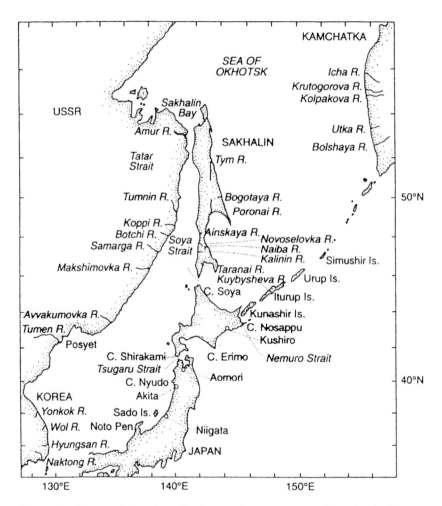

Fig. 4. Far Eastern Asian rivers having anadromous masu salmon in the Korean
Peninsula and USSR. (From Machidori and Kato 1984, with permission)

parasitologist, we defined the so-called *D. latum* in Korea as *D. nihonkaiense*, and also determined the distribution of *D. yonagoense* in Korea in 1996.

The determination of the species of diphyllobothriid cestodes, which is important for the pathological diagnosis of diphyllobothriosis, must be carried out by the following process.

1. Ask the patient if he (she) ate masu salmon.
2. Ask the patient if he (she) traveled abroad (especially in Scandinavia and Russia) and consumed raw fish as the possible infectious source.
3. In therapy after diagnosis, select anthelmintics that do not dissolve the scolex of the worm. Confirm if the evacuated strobila has its scolex. If it has not, repeat the fecal examination after about 30 days and confirm that the treatment is complete.
4. Treat and preserve the evacuated worm by the described and methods process earlier and consult parasitoltololologists for determination of species.

Strategy to Prevent Diphyllobothriosis in Japan

Finally, we suggest four important points for developing a strategy to prevent diphyllobothriosis:

1. International exchange of information on diphyllobothriosis and establishment of a monitoring system.
2. Promotion of ecological study on the natural foci of *Diphyllobothrium* species in the Far East.
3. Determination of the life cycle of *D. nihonkaiense* through interdisciplinary cooperation among the fields of fishery science, marine ecology, etc.
4. Cooperation between food hygiene and public health specialists to educate citizens on diphyllobothriosis through the health promotion strategy of participatory action research.

Acknowledgments. The authors are grateful to Professor H. Ishikura, Sapporo Medical University, Japan, for offering us this precious opportunity to give a lecture in this symposium. We are also grateful to Dr. D.I. Gibson, Natural History Museum, London, United Kingdom, and to the late Dr. L. Margolis, Pacific Biological Station, Nanaimo, Canada.

References

Eguchi S (1926) Studies on *Dibothriocephalus latus*, with a special reference to its life-cycle in Japan (in Japanese). Byorigaku Kiyo 3:1–66

Fukumoto S, Yazaki S, Kamo H, Yamane, Y, Tsuji M (1988) Distinction between *Diphyllobothrium nihonkaiense* and *Diphyllobothrium latum* by immunoelectrophoresis. Jpn J Parasitol 37: 91–95

Fukumoto S, Yazaki S, Nagai D, Takeuchi H, Kamo H, Yamane Y (1987) Comparative studies on soluble protein profiles and isozyme patterns in 3 related species of the genus *Diphyllobothrium*. Jpn J Parasitol 36:222–230

Groot C, Margolis L (1991) Pacific salmon life histories. University of British Columbia Press, Vancouver, Canada

Iijima L (1889) The source of *Bothriocephalus latus* in Japan. Coll Sci Tokyo Imp Univ 2:49–56

Kamo H (1978) Reconsideration on taxonomic status of *Diphyllobothrium latum* (Linnaeus, 1758) in Japan with special regard to species-specific characters. Jpn J Parasitol 27:135–142

Machidori S (1981) The life cycle and the distribution in offshore masu salmon. In: Research report of salmonids fish (in Japanese). Institute of Offshore Fishery, Tokyo

Machidori S, Kato F (1984) Spawning populations and marine life of masu salmon (*Oncorhynchus masou*). Int N Pac Fish Comm Bull 43:11

Tsumura S (1795) Tankai. Edo (Tokyo), Japan

Yamane Y, Kamo H, Bylund G, Wikgren Bo-J P (1986) *Diphyllobothrium nihonkaiense* sp. nov. (Cestoda: Diphyllobothriidae)—revised identification of Japanese broad tapeworm. Shimane J Med Sci 10:29–48

Yamane Y, Shiwaku K, Osaki Y, Okamoto T. (1989) The taxonomic differences of embryonic hooks in *Diphyllobothrium nihonkaiense*, *D. latum* and *D. dendriticum*. Parasitol Res 75:549–553

Histopathological and Immunological Diagnosis for Parasitic Zoonoses

Yukifumi Nawa

Summary. Endemicity of parasitic diseases is largely dependent on the socioeconomic conditions and lifestyle of the population. Rapid improvement of public health conditions together with mass screening and mass treatment has brought about a drastic decrease in the prevalence of soil-transmitted helminthic diseases in Japan. Conversely, imported parasitic diseases are gradually increasing along with the expansion of international activities. In between these changes, domestic foodborne parasitic zoonoses are, although they are still endemic in some areas of Japan, somewhat ignored not only by clinicians but also by parasitologists. Because many domestic foodborne parasitic zoonoses are a kind of visceral larva migrans, these diseases are often misdiagnosed as malignancies. Therefore, although the main focus of this symposium is the internationalization of parasitic diseases, I prefer to focus on the diagnostic procedures of parasitic zoonoses that are currently endemic in Japan.

Key Words: Zoonoses—foodborne diseases—Visceral larva migrans (VLM) — Eosinophilia — IgE — Histopathology — Immunodiagnosis — ELISA — *Paragonimus* — *Gnathostoma* — *Ascaris* — *Dirofilaria* — *Fasciola*—*Toxocara*

Introduction

Soil-transmitted intestinal helminth infections, for example, ascariosis, hookworm disease, and trichuriosis, were previously the most common digestive diseases in Japan. The prevalence of these intestinal helminthiases was, however, drastically reduced by extensive mass

Department of Parasitology, Miyazaki Medical College, Miyazaki 889-1692, Japan

screening and mass treatment, and, more profoundly, by improvement of public health conditions during the past 30 years. Conversely, imported parasitic diseases such as malaria are gradually increasing along with the expansion of such international activities as trading and tourism. The problem is that the drastic decrease in the number of patients with intestinal helminthosis has brought about the misunderstanding that parasitic diseases in general have been eradicated from this country (Nawa 1991). Consequently, some departments and institutes related to parasitic diseases have been restructured to other research fields such as tropical medicine, immunology, and molecular biology. These trends have reduced both manpower in parasitology and diagnostic capability for parasitic diseases. However, on the basis of the cumulative consultations referred to our laboratory for the past 11 years, parasitic diseases seem to be rather increasing in number (Fig. 1), and most of these are foodborne parasitic zoonoses. Because food habits cannot be easily given up, most Japanese still eat "sashimi" and "sushi" with soy sauce, which I call the most important causative "3 S" of Japanese parasitic diseases. Many foodborne parasitic zoonoses in Japan are larva migrans, and thus they

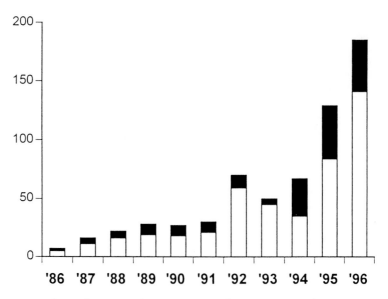

Fig. 1. Numbers of patients whose serum samples were sent to the Department of Parasitology, Miyzaki Medical College, for immunodiagnosis during 1986–1996. *Black bars*, positive; *white bars*, negative

are not detected by fecal egg examination. Once parasite larvae migrate into the visceral organs, the lesions are indistinguishable from those of malignant diseases. In this chapter, I introduce some clues for diagnosis of foodborne parasitic zoonoses in Japan, with special emphasis on histopathological and immunological methods.

Detection of Parasites in Histopathological Specimens

Diagnosis of helminthic diseases is rather easy when worms or eggs are detected in stool or sputum specimens. Even so, an accurate diagnosis could not be reached if a series of laboratory examinations were not properly oriented to determine the pathogens. Patients having intractable diarrhea and body weight loss are often suspected of having a malignancy in the digestive tract, and fecal egg examination is ignored. Although it would be a rare occurrence, such cases may well be severe metagonimosis (Ichiki et al. 1990) (Fig. 2), strongyloidosis (Tanaka et al. 1996), diphyllobothriosis, or, rarely, intestinal capillariosis (Nawa et al. 1988). Because nematode larvae are usually so small, pathologists sometimes overlook the larvae of *Strongyloides stercoralis* (Fig. 3) or *Capillaria*

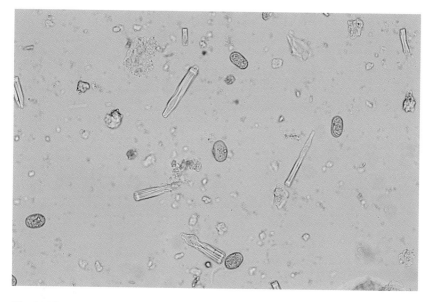

Fig. 2. *Metagonimus yokogawai* eggs found in fecal examination

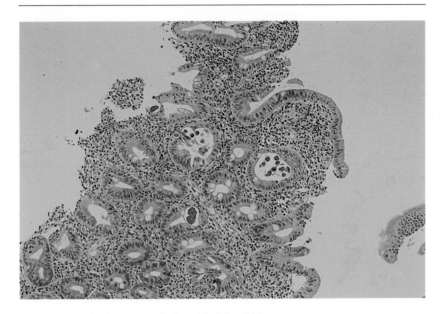

Fig. 3. *Strongyloides stercoralis* found in jejunal biopsy

philippinensis (Fig. 4) in hematoxylin-eosin- (HE-) stained sections of colonic biopsies. Similarly, patients having nodular lesions in the lungs are usually suspected of having lung cancer. When pathologists or laboratory examiners see sputum smears of such patients, they are usually searching for malignant cells, and the presence of *Paragonimus* eggs goes unrecognized (Fig. 5). Bilateral nodular and infiltrating pulmonary lesions with eosinophilia could be diagnosed as allergic granulomatous angiitis. This, however, could also be seen in paragonimosis (Okamoto et al. 1993). Depending on clinical diagnosis, pathologists might pay less attention to the presence of parasite eggs in the specimen.

Regardless of clinical diagnosis, careful pathologists may unexpectedly come across worms or eggs in histopathological sections of biopsied or autopsied specimens. We have had an experience of intraperitoneal granuloma caused by *Paragonimus* that was assumed to be a metastatic lesion of bladder carcinoma (Shimao et al. 1994) (Fig. 6). Intrahepatic cholelithiasis could form around invaded *Paragonimus* (Nabeshima et al. 1991) (Fig. 7) or *Ascaris*.

Sections of worms or parasite eggs can be found in histopathological sections of biopsied specimens suspected to contain worms.

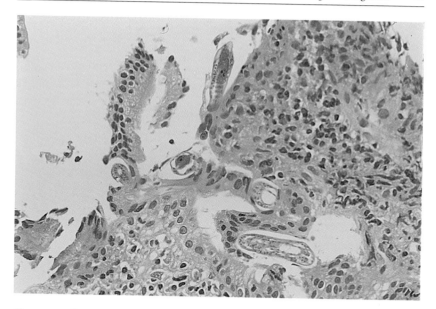

Fig. 4. *Capillaria philippinensis* found in colonic biopsy

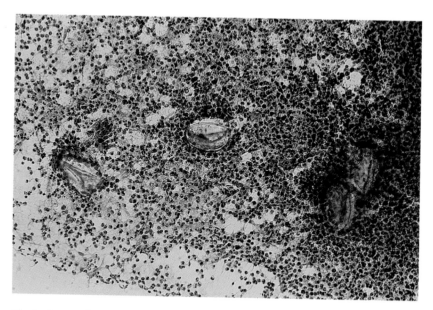

Fig. 5. *Paragonimus westermani* eggs in sputum smear

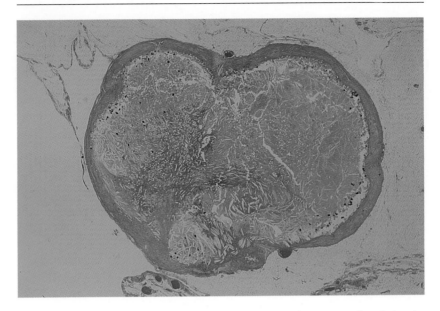

Fig. 6. Nodular lesion containing numerous *Paragonimus* eggs found in the peritoneum

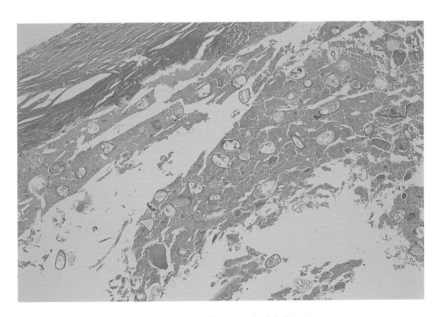

Fig. 7. *Paragonimus* eggs found in intrahepatic cholelithiasis

Gnathostoma (Ogata et al. 1988) and *Spirurina* type X larvae, both of which are known to cause creeping diseases or migratory erythema in the skin, are found and identified easily in sections of biopsied skin (Fig. 8). Still, the detection rate of these parasites in biopsied specimens is less than 20%. Even when patients are suspected to have parasitic diseases because of eosinophilia and elevated IgE, the chance of detecting worms or eggs in biopsied specimens from other sites such as the digestive tract, lung, or liver is assumed to be far lower than in skin. *Dirofilaria* (Suzumiya and Nawa 1990) (Fig. 9), *Spirometra* (Fig. 10), *Toxocara*, *Fasciola*, and other helminths that have migrated into visceral organs can be occasionally found in histopathological sections of biopsy or surgical specimens.

Wherever the site from which the biopsied specimen is obtained, and whatever the causative parasite species, diagnosis is not difficult once worms or eggs are visible because the cut surface of the worms and eggs of each parasite species has unique morphological characteristics useful for identification. A problem occurs when worms or eggs are not detected in biopsied specimens from patients clinically suspected as having parasitic diseases. Eosinophil infiltration in tissue sections could strongly

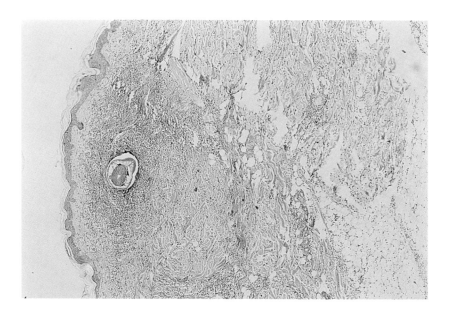

Fig. 8. *Gnathostoma doloresi* larvae found in skin biopsy

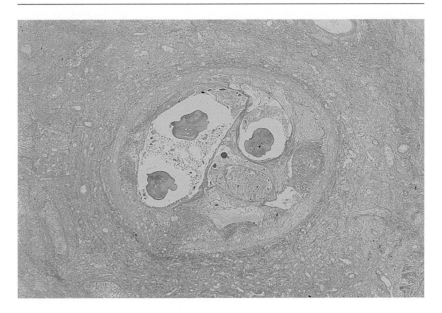

Fig. 9. *Dirofilaria immitis* embolized in pulmonary artery

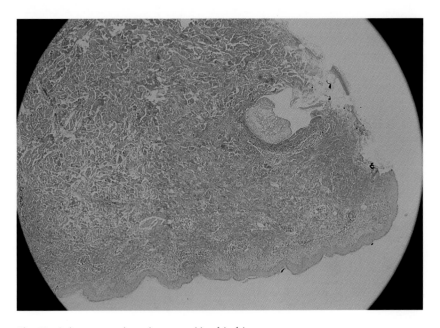

Fig. 10. *Spirometra erinacei-europaei* in skin biopsy

suggest that the inflammatory lesion is caused by parasite infection, although it does not tell anything about the genus or species of such causative pathogens. In such cases, immunoserological methods are the only practical and applicable way to reach diagnosis.

Immunoserological Diagnosis

Recently we have received increasing numbers of referrals from clinicians not only in Miyazaki but also from Kagoshima, Kumamoto, Fukuoka, and other places in Japan (Maruyama et al. 1996) (Fig. 11). Most cases referred to our laboratory were patients having eosinophilia and elevated total IgE of unknown etiology. These patients having eosinophilia/hyper-IgE frequently had lung or liver lesions, but eggs and worms were rarely detected in the stool, sputum, or biopsied specimens. When sera from such patients reach us, we usually use a multiple dot-ELISA (enzyme-linked immunosorbent assay) test for the first step of screening. In our system, crude somatic extracts of 12 different helminths are precoated on nitrocellulose membrane (Fig. 12). The membrane is incubated with ×200 diluted patient's serum, washed, and then incubated with horse radish peroxidase- (HRP) labeled rabbit antihuman IgG antibody. After wash-

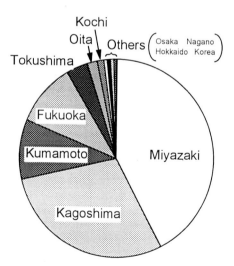

Fig. 11. Geographic distributions of serum samples referred for immunodiagnosis to the Department of Parasitology, Miyazaki Medical College, during 1996

病院　　　　科　　　　　　　　先生侍史

Multiple-dot ELISA Test for Parasitic Diseases

Date :

Patient's name :　　　　　　　　　　Age :　　　Sex :

Hospital :　　　　　　　　　Corresponding Dr.:

Address :　　　　　　　　　　Phone :

FAX :

Sample examined :

Other remarks :

	◯	(Positive cont. for reagent)
Dirofilaria immitis : Di	◯ ◯	Pw : *Paragonimus westermanii*
Toxocara canis : Tc	◯ ◯	Pm : *Paragonimus miyazakii*
Ascaris suum : As	◯ ◯	Fh : *Fasciola hepatica*
Anisakis simplex : Asx	◯ ◯	Cs : *Clonorchis sinensis*
Gnathostoma doloresi : Gd	◯ ◯	Se : *Spirometra erinacei*
Strongyloides ratti : Sr	◯ ◯	Cc : *Cysticercus cellulosae*

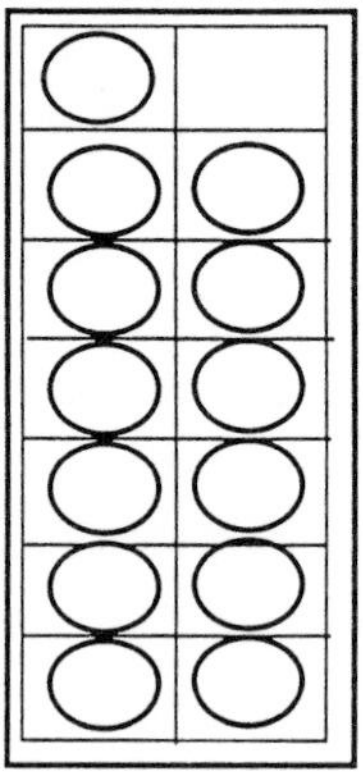

Results :

Comments :

Date of Diagnosis :

Consultant :

〒889-16 宮崎県宮崎郡清武町木原5200
宮崎医科大学寄生虫学教室
TEL:0985-85-0990(直通)　学内内線: 2159
FAX:0985-84-3887

Deprtment of Parasitology
Miyazaki Medical College
Kiyotake, Miyazaki 889-16
Phone: 0985-85-0990
F A X: 0985-84-3887

Fig. 12. Schematic diagram of multiple-dot ELISA (enzyme-linked immunosorbent assay) used in the Department of Parasitology, Miyazaki Medical College

ing, the membrane is incubated with a substrate solution containing H_2O_2 as the substrate and 4-chloro-1-naphthol as the chromogen. Diagnosis is made by visual scoring (Fig. 13a). The whole process of screening by multiple dot-ELISA requires only 3h or less. If a patient's serum reacts with multiple parasite antigens in the multiple dot-ELISA, we examine further the reactivity of the patient's serum to the suspected antigens by a double immunodiffusion test in agarose (Ouchterlony's method) (Fig. 13b) or by combinations of binding and binding-inhibition ELISA.

Cumulative data using these immunoserological tests revealed that about 30% of eosinophilic patients referred to our laboratory were diagnosed as having parasitic diseases. Particularly, the percentage of seropositive cases for parasitic diseases rose to about 70% when patients had eosinophilia of 20% or greater associated with lung or liver lesions (Maruyama et al. 1996) (Fig. 14). In Kyushu, paragonimosis was the most common disease, followed by gnathostomosis, fasciolosis, and visceral larva migrans caused by *Ascaris suum* and other parasite species such as *Toxocara*. The traditional custom of the residents in Kyushu of eating the flesh of freshwater fish and wild animals is the main reason for the endemicity of these foodborne parasitic zoonoses.

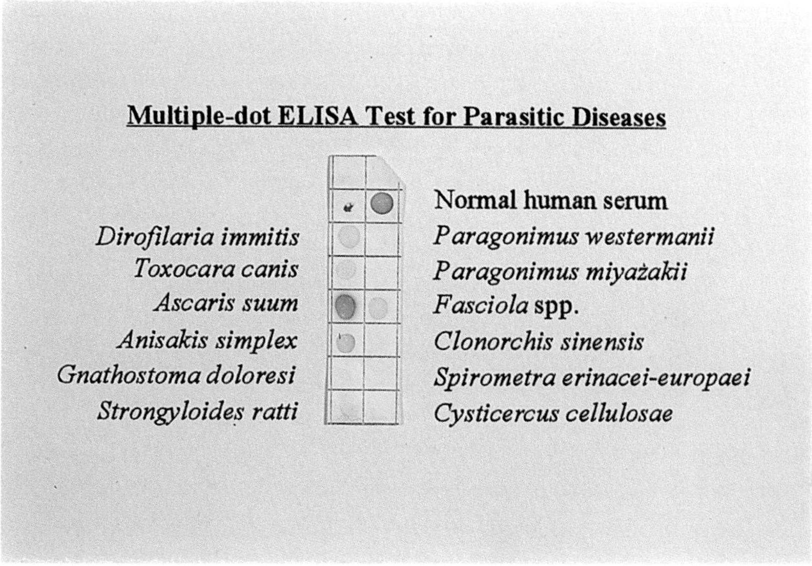

Fig. 13. a The multiple-dot ELISA. This sample is strongly positive against *Ascaris suum* with some cross-reaction to other nematode antigens. **b** Using Ouchterlony's double immunodiffusion test in agarose, the sample shows positive reaction against *A. suum. Al, A. lumbricoides; Asx, Anisakis simplex; As, A. suum; Tc, Toxocara canis*

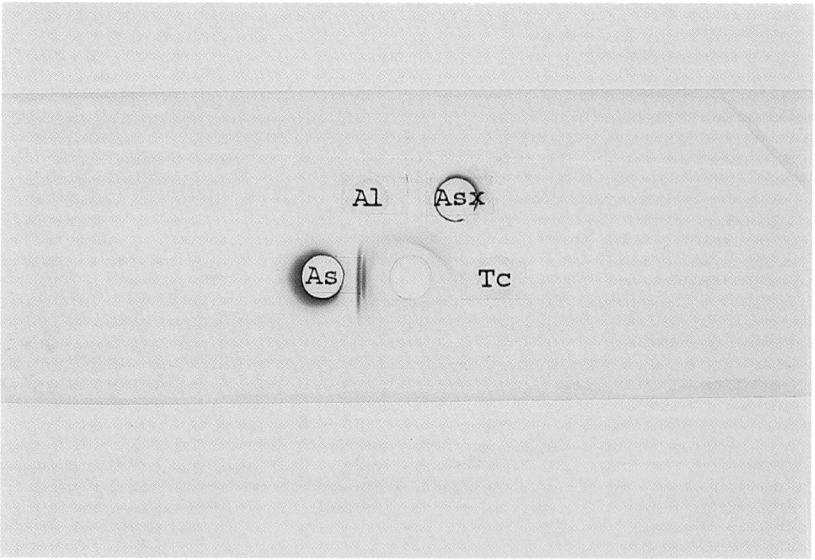

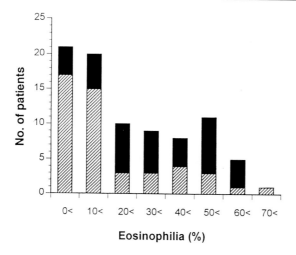

Fig. 14. Correlation between the degree of eosinophilia (%) and the number of positive cases for parasitic diseases by immunodiagnosis. *Black bars*, positive; *shaded bars*, negative

Problems and Future Tasks

The results reported here as well as those of others suggest that both domestic and imported parasitic diseases seem to be increasing in number. The most serious problems of parasitic diseases is that nationwide surveillance for each parasitic disease has never been done properly. This occurs because, except for malaria and some other protozoan infections, most parasitic diseases are never considered as a serious public health issue nowadays. The worst problem is that the number of departments or laboratories capable of dealing with the diagnosis of parasitic diseases is drastically decreasing along with the recent restructuring of universities and research institutes.

Concerning histopathological examinations for parasitic diseases, many experts in this field have passed away or retired and their skills seem not to have been transferred to the next generation. Many important reference specimens seem to have been lost or dispersed. Because histopathological specimens are usually examined first by pathologists, the Japanese Society of Pathology should, in conjunction with the Japanese Society of Parasitology, consider establishing a training course or reference textbook for parasitological examinations in biopsied specimens.

Another serious problem is that immunoserological diagnosis for parasitic diseases depends entirely on the voluntary work of individual researchers. Although various immunodiagnostic methods have been developed by Japanese parasitologists, regretfully these methods have never been standardized. Even now, neither standard antigens nor standard positive sera are available in Japan. This urgent problem should be solved by the Japanese Society of Parasitology.

In conclusion, establishment of parasitic disease reference laboratories with training courses would be a desirable way to maintain and expand the diagnistic capability for parasitic diseases.

References

Ichiki Y, Tanaka T, Haraguchi Y, et al (1990) A case of severe metagonimosis with abdominal symptoms. Jpn J Parasitol 39:72–74

Maruyama H, Noda S, Nawa Y (1996) Emerging problems of parasitic diseases in southern Kyushu, Japan. Jpn J Parasitol 45:192–200

Nabeshima K, Inoue T, Sekiya R, et al (1991) Intrahepatic paragonimosis—a case report. Jpn J Parasitol 40:296–300

Nawa Y (1991) Helminthic diseases—some clues for the diagnosis and treatment based on the recent experience in Japan. Asian Med J 34:83–88

Nawa Y, Imai J, Abe T, et al (1988) A case report of intestinal capillariosis—the second case found in Japan. Jpn J Parasitol 2:113–118

Ogata K, Imai J, Nawa Y (1988) Three confirmed and five suspected human cases of Gnathostoma doloresi infection found in Miyazaki Prefecture, Kyushu. Jpn J Parasitol 37:358–364

Okamoto M, Miyake Y, Shouji S, et al (1993) A case of severe paragonimosis miyazakii with lung and skin lesions showing massive egg production in sputum and faeces. Jpn J Parasitol 42:429–433

Shimao Y, Koono M, Ochiai A, et al (1994) A case report of intraperitoneal granuloma due to occult infection with Paragonimus sp. Jpn J Parasitol 43:315–317

Suzumiya J, Nawa Y (1990) Three cases of pulmonary dirofilariosis found in Miyazaki Prefecture. Jpn J Parasitol 39:67–71

Tanaka S, Okumura Y, Maruyama H, et al (1996) A case of overwhelming strongyloidosis cured by repeated administration of ivermectin. Jpn J Parasitol 45:152–156

The Pathology of Cerebral Malaria

Masamichi Aikawa

Summary. Blockage of cerebral microvessels by *Plasmodium falciparum*-infected erythrocytes appears to be the principal cause of the pathology of cerebral malaria. Knobs on infected erythrocytes act as the focal junctions of cell contact to endothelial cells. The knobs are, therefore, important in blockage of the microvascular lumen and in ensuring pathological changes in cerebral tissues. Immunological events might also play an important role in the pathogenesis of cerebral malaria. It is important to assess the candidate malaria vaccines now in development, not only for their efficacy in reducing blood parasitemia but also for any effects they have to increase or decrease the sequestration of infected erythrocytes in the brain and the attendant pathology.

Key Words: Pathogenesis of cerebral malaria—Cytoadherence proteins—Malaria antigens—Capillary obstruction

Introduction

According to a report from the World Health Organization (WHO), in any given year there are, worldwide, 300–500 million patients with malaria. Of these, 1.5–3 million will die annually. This high mortality rate is in large part caused by the appearance of strains of *Plasmodium falciparum* that are resistant to the antimalarial drugs currently in use and the concomitant evolution of strains of mosquitoes that are resistant to available insecticides. Environmental changes such as the mass movement of whole populations to malaria endemic regions and the elevation of global temperatures have led to outbreaks of malaria in certain geo-

Research Institute of Medical Sciences, Tokai University, Bohseidai, Isehara, Kanagawa 259-1193, Japan

graphic areas. In 1996, about 120 cases of malaria were reported in Japan. These infections may be the result of visits by Japanese travelers to malaria endemic regions as well as foreign visitors to Japan coming from such areas. Among the different types of malaria, the one of greatest concern is falciparum malaria, an often fatal affliction. The falciparum form of malaria causes severe symptoms, particularly cerebral malaria. This latter manifestation of the disease is estimated to directly lead to the deaths of 20%–50% of infected patients.

Cerebral malaria is defined as an acute, diffuse, and symmetrical encephalopathy in patients with falciparum malaria and should be confined to patients with demonstrable asexual forms of *P. falciparum* who are in coma; other causes of encephalopathy, such as bacterial, fungal, or viral meningoencephalopathies, drug intoxication, head injury, eclampsia, hypoglycemia, and cerebrovascular accident, should be excluded. The duration of fever, the exact duration and speed of onset of coma, occurrence of convulsions, and the use of antimalarials should be carefully questioned. In Africa, cerebral malaria is unusual in adults because immunity is obtained in childhood through repeated malaria infection. However, in young children presenting in coma and showing *P. falciparum* in their blood cells, cerebral malaria is indicated.

Possible factors contributing to the development of cerebral malaria include the blockage of cerebral microvessels by parasitized red blood cells, deposition of immune complexes in brain capillaries, reduced humoral of cell-mediated immune responses, action of tumor necrosis factor, and nitric oxide, in addition to other factors (Aikawa 1988). Among these, the blockage of cerebral microvessels has been considered to be the major factor in the pathogenesis of cerebral malaria.

Of the countries of the world where malaria is a major problem, Myanmar is a good example, with about 800000 cases of malaria annually. In Myanmar cases, *P. falciparum* is the major cause. Similarly, cerebral malaria cases are often seen in Cambodia, Thailand, and Vietnam. Using light and electron microscopy and an immunoperoxidase technique, we have examined brain tissue specimens from patients who died of cerebral malaria (Oo et al. 1987; Riganti et al. 1980; Pongponratn et al. 1991; Aikawa et al. 1990). Based on our pathological findings of cerebral malaria patients, the possible pathogenesis of human cerebral malaria is discussed here.

Rodent models of cerebral malaria are not discussed because the pathology of cerebral malaria occurring in rodents is different from that in humans with cerebral malaria. There is no blockage of cerebral microvessels in rodent models of cerebral malaria. The knobs on *P. falciparum*-infected erythrocytes are important for the development of human cerebral malaria, but, rodent parasites do not cause formation of knobs in infected erythrocytes (Aikawa 1988). However, there have been many reports on cerebral malaria pathogenesis based on rodent models, so one should be careful when interpreting such data.

The Pathology of Human Cerebral Malaria

On autopsy, the brain of patients who have died of cerebral malaria is edematous, heavy, and has broadened and flattened gyri. There may be grooving of the uncinated and cingulate gyri and of the cerebrellar tonsils. The vessels of the arachnoid are congested, giving the so-called pink brain. The cut surface shows selective congestion and hemorrhage of the white matter. Light microscopy shows cerebral microvessels filled with parasitized erythrocytes (PRBC) mixed with uninfected erythrocytes (Oo et al. 1987; Riganti et al. 1990; Pongponratn et al. 1991; Aikawa et al. 1990) (Fig. 1). Occasional inflammatory cells are present adjacent to microvessels engorged with PRBC. Infected erythrocytes in small and medium-sized arteries are seen attached to the endothelial cells; however, they rarely block the lumen of these vessels. Ring hemorrhages (Fig. 2) and Duck's granulomas are lesions in the brains of patients with cerebral malaria who survive for at least 10 days of clinical malaria. Necrotic arterioles and capillaries are present in the center of these hemorrhages (Oo et al. 1987). Duck's granulomas are areas of softening, demyelinization, and glial proliferation.

Electron microscopy demonstrates multiple electron-dense knobs protruding from the membrane of PRBC in the microvessels. Scanning electron microscopy shows that the knobs are evenly distributed over the erythrocyte membrane (Fig. 3). These electron-dense knobs form focal junctions with the endothelial cells and adjacent erythrocytes, causing the obstruction of cerebral microvessels (Fig. 4). Immunocytochemistry shows linear staining of *P. falciparum* antigens along the walls of the microvessels (Aikawa et al. 1990). IgG and IgM are also present along these microvessels.

Because the knobs on PRBC that form their focal junctions to endothelial cells and other erythrocytes appear to be important in mediating

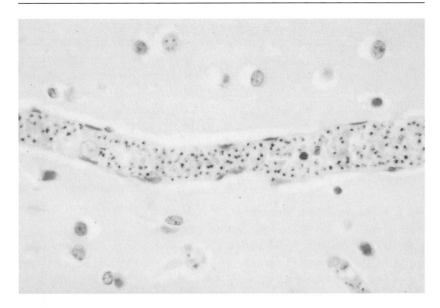

Fig. 1. Light photomicrograph of cerebral microvessels filled with parasitized erythrocytes mixed with uninfected erythrocytes

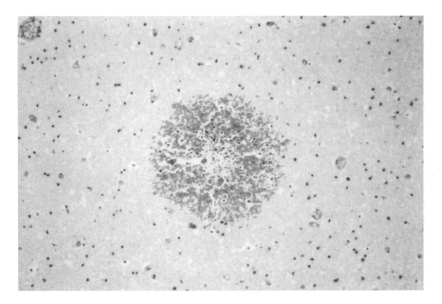

Fig. 2. Light photomicrograph of a ring hemorrhage

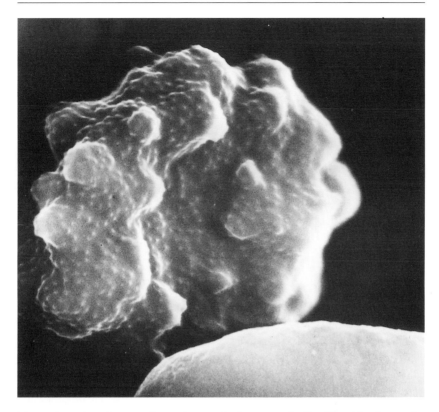

Fig. 3. Scanning electron photomicrograph shows evenly distributed knobs on the erythrocyte membrane

blockage of microvascular lumens, the role of knob proteins in cerebral malaria has been studied. Electron microscopy reveals electron-dense materials (EDM) within the cytoplasm of *P. falciparum* that are often associated with the parasite membrane (Aikawa et al. 1987). The EDM are also seen associated with unit membrane-bounded Mauler's clefts in PRBC. These EDM have the same density and appearance as the material located under knobs at the erythrocyte membrane. Immunoelectron microscopy shows the association of ankyrin with the membrane of clefts (Fujioka and Aikawa 1996; Atkinson and Aikawa 1990). The presence of ankyrin on the membrane of clefts indicates that some clefts are derived from the erythrocyte membrane because ankyrin is known to be present on the erythrocyte membrane. Thus, the parasite-derived EDM appears to

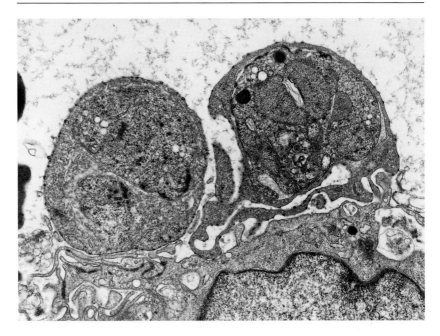

Fig. 4. Electron photomicrograph showing infected erythrocytes binding to the endothelial cells by knobs

be transported from the parasite plasmalemma to the erythrocyte membrane via Mauler's clefts in the erythrocyte cytoplasm.

Since Kilejian first reported histidine-rich knob-associated protein (HRP) in 1979, many investigators have described the expression and gene sequence of this molecule. As the presence of HRP in knobs is an important factor in knob formation, we investigated whether a histidine analog, 2-fluoro-L-histidine, might affect the formation of knobs (Aikawa et al. 1987). When the parasites were cultivated in the presence of 2-fluoro-L-histidine, the amount of EDM in the parasitophorous vacuole increased. We also noted that the density of this EDM increased with increasing levels of 2-fluoro-L-histidine. 2-Fluoro-L-histidine also increased the amount and density of EDM associated with Mauler's clefts in the host erythrocyte cytoplams. As the concentration of 2-fluoro-L-histidine increased, the number of infected cells having knobs and the number of knobs per cell both decreased. Quantitative analyses of the surface area of EDM associated with the parasitophorous vacuole mem-

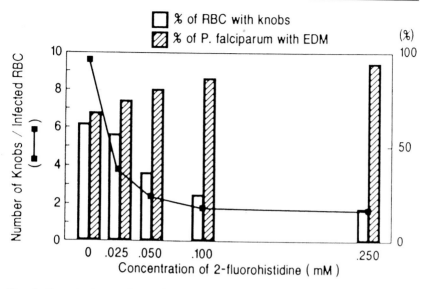

Fig. 5. Quantitative analysis of the effects of 2-fluoro-L-histidine on knobs and electron-dense materials (EDM) associated with the parasitophorous vacuole

brane, percentage of PRBC having knobs, and number of knobs per infected cell at different concentrations of 2-fluoro-L-histidine are shown in Fig. 5. It appears that this histidine analog blocks export of EDM from the parasite to the knobs and thereby affects knob formation. Thus, this analog might be used for prevention of adhesion of infected cells to the endothelial cells and eventually the prevention of the development of cerebral malaria.

At least six malaria proteins (PfHRP1, PfHRP2, PfHRP3, PfEMP1, PfEMP2, PfEMP3) have been identified in the surface of *P. falciparum*-infected erythrocytes (Fujioka and Aikawa 1996) (HRP, histidine-rich protein; EMP, erythrocyte membrane protein). All of these, with the exception of PfHRP2, are localized in knobs (Fig. 6). PfHRP1 and PfHRP3 appear to relate to the knob structure itself. Immunoelectron microscopy demonstrates the presence of PfHRP1 and PfHRP3 within the knobs. PfHRP2 secretes to the outside from the infected erythrocytes. PfEMP1 and PfEMP2 do not contain histidine. PfEMP1 is an antigenically diverse 200- to 350-kDa surface protein of PRBC and seems to be one of the major cytoadherent proteins, mediating the adherence of PRBC to microvascu-

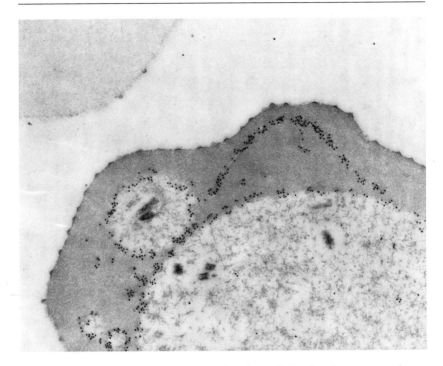

Fig. 6. Immunoelectron photomicrographs show EMP1 (erythrocyte membrane protein) on the surface of knobs

lar endothelial cells in cerebral malaria patients. This protein had been shown, in vitro, to mediate the adherence of PRBC to purified platelet glycoprotein IV (CD 36), thrombospondin (TSP), and intracellular adhesion molecule-1 (ICAM-1).

PfEMP2 is polymorphic in size, 250- to 300-kDa in different isolates, and has been localized in the parasitophorous vacuole of the schizont, within membrane-bound vesicles in the erythrocyte cytoplasm, and in association with knobs and the inner face of the erythrocyte membrane covering the knobs. PfEMP2 interacts with the 80-kDa membrane cytoskeletal phosphoprotein band 4.1. PfEMP3 is a newly isolated surface antigen that has been located on the erythrocyte membrane. Knobless strains of *P. falciparum* carry deletions of the gene encoding PfEMP3. PfEMP3 may be involved in knob formation, and it is suspected that it interacts with a protein or proteins of the erythrocyte cytoskeleton

(Atkinson and Aikawa 1990; Kilejian et al. 1991). The exact role of the antigen in cytoadherence remains unclear.

Pf155/RESA is a ring-infected erythrocyte surface antigen that has been localized specifically in the micronemes of merozoites. This molecule is translocated to the erythrocyte membrane or cytoskeleton from micronemes of merozoites that have newly invaded the erythrocyte. This molecule is a spectrin-binding protein that forms a complex with actin, spectrin, and band 4.1.

Antigenically Variant PfEMP1 Molecules Are Encoded by *var* Genes

Important papers have recently been published that show that *P. falciparum* contains a large family of genes (*var*) encoding antigenically variant molecules that modulate the adhesive properties of infected erythrocytes. Proteins encoded by the *var* family belong to a large super-family (DBL) that includes proteins involved in erythrocyte invasion. The *var* genes are highly diverse and are present on multiple chromosomes at a copy of 50–150 per parasite. An individual *var* gene encodes 200- to 350-kDa molecules with highly variable extracellular regions that contain homologous to cystine-rich binding domains of certain erythrocyte-binding proteins such as *Plasmodium vivax* Duffy antigen-binding protein and *P. falciparum* EBA 175. PfEMP1 of the MC parasite is encoded by a *var* gene: antibody raised against peptide sequences from the MC *var* open reading frame recognized PfEMP1 at the knobs, blocking adherence of the infected cells to CD36, and agglutinated MC-infected erythrocytes in a strain-specific manner. Rapid switching in the antigenic and cytoadherence properties of the infected erythrocytes is correlated with switches in the transcription of *var* genes. These findings imply that individual parasites probably express on, or at most on a few, *var* genes.

The antigenically variant adhesive molecules encoded by the *var* genes have the potential to bind a wide range of endothelial cell receptors, including ICAM-1, CD36, and TSP. These diverse binding properties are consistent with the need for the parasite to sequester within tissue vacuolar beds while maintaining the ability to vary the antigenic properties of PfEMP1. Switches in PfEMP1 expression may not only affect the phenotype of a parasite strain but may change its sequestration properties and virulence.

Mechanism of PRBC Adhesion to Endothelial Cell Receptors

Recent studies of the molecular basis of sequestration in vitro and in vivo have shown that adhesion of PRBC is caused by a receptor-mediated interaction of ligands on the PRBC membrane with host receptors on the surface of vascular endothelial cells. PRBC can bind to at least three major host cell-surface receptors, such as ICAM-1, CD36, and TSP. A role for E-section and vascular cell adhesion molecule-1 (VCAM-1) has also been proposed concerning the surface receptors of PRBC. The levels of ICAM-1 expression are highly correlated with the degree of parasite sequestration in brain capillaries.

The first candidate receptor model is ICAM-1 (Fujioka and Aikawa 1996). Studies with COS cell transfectants and human umbilical vein endothelium (HUVEC) have shown that ICAM-1 is an endothelial cell receptor for PRBC. PRBC bound onto purified ICAM-1-coated plastic surfaces. In addition, PRBC were capable of binding to COS cells transfected with the cDNA of ICAM-1 and also to cytokine-activated HUVEC. In patients who died of cerebral malaria, the postmortem brain showed positive staining for ICAM-1 along the microvascular endothelium, which was packed with PRBC cytoadhering to the endothelium. During physiological blood flow through the brain microvasculature, random contacts may occur between PRBC and endothelial cells. Endothelial "activation" leads to upregulation of specific surface receptor(s), e.g., ICAM-1, and this molecule may initiate adhesion of PRBC to the microvascular endothelium.

The molecular basis for adhesion of PRBC to ICAM-1 is not well known, although domain 1 has been identified as a binding site for PRBC. ICAM-1 as a ligand for the leukocyte integrins, lymphocyte function-associated antigen-1 (LFA-1:CD11a/CD18) and Mac-1(CD11b/CD 18), has also served as a receptor for the major group of human rhinoviruses (HRV). Monoclonal antibodies (MAbs) that inhibit binding of LFA-1 and HRV to ICAM-1 have no effect on PRBC binding to purified ICAM-1 being spatially distinct from the recognition sites for LFA-1 and HRV. It has been postulated that domain 2 of ICAM-1, which plays an essential role in ICAM-1 conformation, might also be directly involved in the binding site. PfEMP1 is, in fact, the ligand most likely to mediate the adhesion of PRBC to the ICAM-1 and CD36 receptors expressed on the endothelium because antigenically variant PfEMP1 molecules are encoded in *var* genes. The proteins in the superfamily encoded in the *var* gene have the potential to mediate binding to various receptors on the endothelial cells in brain microvessels.

The second candidate for a receptor model is CD36. As with ICAM-1, PRBC bound to purified CD36-coated plastic and also bound to COS cells tranfected with cDNA encoding CD36. The anti-CD36 monoclonal antibodies OKM5 and OKM8 inhibit PRBC cytoadherence in vitro. Nakamura et al. (1992) reported localization of the PRBC receptor for CD36 on the electron-dense knob protrusions of the PRBC surface. Ockenhouse et al. (1992) also confirmed that the human CD36 epitope defined by MAbs OKM5 and OKM8 forms the erythrocyte-binding site, measured by antibody inhibition and antiidiotype antibody mimicry of a CD36-binding domain.

The third candidate model is TSP, a multifunctional glycoprotein that is synthesized by many adherent cell types, including endothelium. PRBC bound to TSP immobilized on plastic. Soluble TSP or polyclonal antibodies against TSP inhibited the adhesion of PRBC to immobilized TSP in vitro. Although the PRBC receptor(s) for TSP have also been demonstrated on the electron-dense knob protrusions of the PRBC surface, other studies have found no inhibition of adhesion with anti-TSP antibodies. TSP was not detected on the highly cytoadherent C32 amelanotic melanoma cell line, and the levels of expression of TSP were not clearly elevated in cerebral venules packed with PRBC. TSP may not be a primary receptor for adherence.

There was a difference in some *P. falciparum* clones or isolates in their ability to bind to different receptors on the cell surface. A *P. falciparum* clone exhibited the ability to switch antigenic and cytoadherence phenotypes, which were selected for binding to C32 melanoma cells or HUVEC. These results, and recent findings such as the antigenically variant PfEMP1 molecules encoded by the *var* gene, suggest that falciparum malaria parasites have the capacity to utilize multiple cytoadherence receptors, and that several families of cytoadherent molecules might be participating in a cascade of binding events leading to PRBC adherence.

The Knob Structure as Revealed by Atomic Force Microscopy

The atomic force microscope (AFM) was developed by Binnig, Quate, and Gerber in 1986. The principle of the AFM is as follows: when a fine needle (a diamond or silicon nitride) that is attached to a cantilevered spring passes over the surface of a specimen, it is deflected by van der Waals forces generated between the atoms of the needle tip and the atoms of the specimen. The deflection force is converted to a surface image of the specimen by computer. The major advantage that the AFM holds over conventional transmission and scanning electron microscopes is that biological specimens do not require fixation and dehydration before they can be examined; in other words, unfixed specimens in a fluid environment can be examined in the AFM. Thus, the long-held hope of biologists of being able to study living cells at high resolution has been realized.

We have begun to utilize the AFM in studies of malaria (Aikawa et al. 1996). Studies using the transmission electron microscope (TEM) have shown that cytoadherence of infected erythrocytes to capillary endothelium involves membrane knobs on the red cell surface. These knobs have now been studied with the AFM to determine if there might be some unrecognized factor that plays a role in cytoadherence. Human erythrocytes infected with *P. falciparum* (Indochina-1/CDC strain) were suspended in phosphate-buffered saline (PBS) and, without further treatment, a drop was placed on a stub coated with polypyrrole and examined in a Digital Instrument AFM (Santa Barbara, CA) atomic force microscope. To determine localized surface charge, the surface potential microscope (SPM), a component of the Digital Instrument Nanoscope III system, was used.

TEM has established that the knobs on fixed, infected erythrocytes are conical and measure about 100 nm at the base and 60 nm in height. Section analysis in the AFM revealed that instead of a single protrusion, there are two distinct peaks in each knob, corresponding to binary subunits; the larger is about 60 nm at its base and the smaller about 40 nm. In other words, instead of consisting of a single protrusion, as appears to be the case in chemically fixed specimens, each knob comprises a pair of subunits (Fig. 7). These paired protrusions are even more distinct when the stage is tilted 45°. Clearly, the true architecture of the membrane knobs is effaced by fixation.

Surface potential spectroscopy showed that the knobs are positively charged (+20 mV), although the remainder of the surface of PRBC has a negative charge. The reversal of charge that characterizes the knobs might be caused by the aggregation of malarial antigens at the knob surface; if such antigens have a net negative charge of sufficient magnitude, it might prevail locally over the normally positive charge of the erythrocyte membrane. Because the luminal plasma membrane of endothelial cells has a

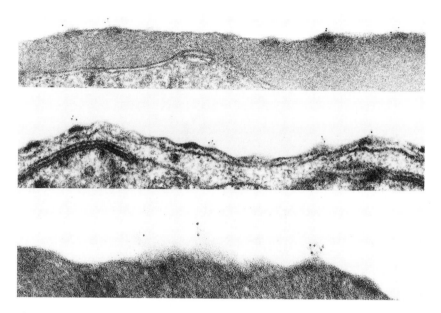

Fig. 7. Immunoelectron micrograph of *P. falciparum* infected erythrocytes. Gold particles indicate the location of PfEMP1 molecules

negative charge, the differences in charge between the erythrocyte knob and endothelial plasmalemma might be involved in cytoadherence between the two. Electrical interaction conceivably could slow the passage of infected erythrocytes over the endothelium sufficiently to permit chemical bonds to form between knob antigens and endothelial receptors, leading to firm cytoadherence.

A similar electrically based phenomenon may be operative at another stage of the malaria disease process. During erythrocyte invasion by merozoites, the positively charged apical end of the parasite appears to be attracted to the negatively charged erythrocyte plasma membrane (Fujioka and Aikawa 1996). This initial electrical event is succeeded by chemical bonding.

The significant findings of this study are that (1) knobs have a more complex morphology than heretofore has been recognized, and (2) knobs have a positive electrical charge, whereas the remainder of the erythrocyte surface has a negative charge. Each of these factors might be central to the phenomenon of cytoadherence in malaria. The importance of electrical phenomena in biological processes is emphasized by the AFM. A therapy based on disruption of knob electrical charge may be a key to the prevention of cerebral malaria. The AFM and SPM can be used to monitor the effectiveness of new medication by examination of unfixed, infected erythrocytes.

Predictors of Survival in Cerebral Malaria Patients

In critically ill patients with a variety of disorders, gastric intramucosal pH has been reported to predict the risk for massive gastrointestinal bleeding, sepsis, multiple organ failure, and outcome. Cerebral malaria is a rapidly progressive encephalopathy with mortality as great as 50% with standard antimalarial therapy. Therefore, improved means for monitoring patients with cerebral malaria are urgently needed. Wilairatana et al. recently reported that measurements of gastric intramucosal pH on admission and again 6h later have a high specificity for prediction in patients with cerebral malaria (84.2% and 100%, respectively).

Intramucosal pH values were significantly lower at the time of admission in cerebral malaria patients who died than in those who survived. Striking differences in patient mortality were evident with respect to the pattern of change from admission to 6-h values for gastric intramucosal pH. Patients in whom therapeutic measures failed to correct a low admission gastric intramucosal pH had the highest mortality rate (80%), whereas survival dramatically improved in those patients whose gastric intramucosal pH returned to normal during the first 6h (mortality, 0%). A pathological study of tissues from patients who had died of cerebral malaria showed extensive sequestration of parasitized erythrocytes in microvessels of the gastric mucosa, suggesting that impaired blood flow had contributed to the development of severe hypoxia in the mucosa. Tissue oxygenation remains difficult to assess clinically, so that it is important to find appropriate monitoring tools that may be correlated with survival. The rapid and simple measurement of gastric intramucosal pH may provide a useful, non-invasive means of identifying those patients at the greatest risk of death and of monitoring the effects of therapeutic interventions in patients with cerebral malaria.

Another method predicting the prognosis of cerebral malaria patients is biopsy of subcutaneous tissues (Nagasawa et al. 1995). As discussed previously, a prominent feature of cerebral malaria is PRBC sequestration within cerebral microvessels. Nakazawa et al. have recently reported the presence of PRBC sequestration in subcutaneous tissues biopsied from comatose patients with cerebral malaria and suggested sequestration in cerebral microvessels, although it was not possible to examine the patients' brains to determine the presence of PRBC sequestration. When rhesus monkeys with cerebral malaria were examined, Nakano et al. found PRBC sequestration in both cerebral and subcutaneous tissues, and the rate of sequestration was similarly high in both tissues. A good correlation of PRBC sequestration rate in the brain and subcutaneous tissues indicated that biopsy of subcutaneous tissues may be useful for the determination of the severity and prognosis of cerebral malaria.

Correlation between severe malaria and blood levels of nitric oxide (NO) has been controversial (Taylor-Robinson 1996). Clark and Rpclett proposed that NO might play a significant role in the development of coma in patients with cerebral malaria, whereas Grau and Kossodo reported that NO is not likely to be involved in the actual process of neurovascular damage during cerebral malaria. Recently, Weinberg et al. reported that children in Tanzania with cerebral malaria had the lowest levels of NO, while infected children with no symptoms had levels elevated above normal. This suggests that NO might help protect against the most severe forms of the disease. Future research is obviously needed concerning the role of NO in cerebral malaria.

Acknowledgments. This work was partially supported by a grant-in-aid for scientific research from the Japanese Ministry of Education, Science, Sports and Culture and a research grant from the U.S. National Institutes of Health (AI-135827).

References

Aikawa M (1988) Human cerebral malaria. Am J Trop Med Hyg 39:3–10

Aikawa M, Uni S, Andrutis AT, Kirk KL, Cohen LA, Howard RJ (1987) In: Chang KP, Anf Snary D (eds) Host-parasite cellular and molecular interactions in protozoal infections. Springer, Heidelberg, pp 297–306

Aikawa M, Iseki M, Barnwell J, Taylor D, Oo MM (1990) The pathology of human cerebral malaria. Am J Trop Med Hyg 43(suppl):43:30–37

Aikawa M, Kanamura K, Shiroishi S, Matsumoto Y, Arwati H, Torri M, Ito Y, Takeuchi T, Tandler B (1996) Membrane knobs of unfixed *Plasmodium falciparum* infected erythrocytes: new findings as revealed by atomic force microscopy and surface potential spectroscopy, Exp Parasitol 84:339–343

Atkinson CT, Aikawa M (1990) Ultrastructure of malaria-infected erythrocytes, Blood Cells (NY) 16:351–368

Fujioka H, Aikawa M, (1996) The molecular basis of pathogenesis of cerebral malaria. Microb Pathog 20:63–72

Kilejian A, Rashid MA, Aikawa M, Aji T, Yang YF (1991) Selective association of a fragment of the knob protein with spectrin, actin and the red cell membrane. Mol Biochem Parasitol 44:175–182

Nagasawa S, Looareesuwan S, Fujioka H, Pongponratrn E, Luk KD, Rabbege JR, Aikawa M (1995), A correlation between sequestrated parasitized erythrocytes in subcutaneous tissues and cerebral malaria, Am J Trop Med Hyg 53:544–546

Nakamura K, Hasler T, Morehead RJ, Howard RJ, Aikawa M (1992) *Plasmodium falciparum* erythrocyte receptor(s) for CD36 and thrombospondin are restricted knobs on the erythrocyte surface, J Histochem Cytochem., 40:1419–1422

Ockenhouse CF, Tegoshi T, Maeno Y, Benjamin C, Ho M, Aikawa M, Lobb RR (1992) Human vascular endothelial cell adhesion receptors for *Plasmodium falciparum*-infected erythrocytes. J Exp Med 176:1183–1189

Oo MM, Aikawa M, Than T, Aya TM, Myint PT, Igarashi I, Schoene WC (1987) Human cerebral malaria: a pathological study. J Neuropathol Exp Neurol 46:223–231

Pongponratn E, Riganti M, Punpoowong B, Aikawa M (1991) Microvascular sequestration of parasitized erythrocytes in human falciparum malaria: a pathological study. Am J Trop Med Hyg 44:168–175

Riganti M, Pongponratn E, Tegoshi T, Looareesuwan S, Punwoowong B, Aikawa M (1990) Human cerebral malaria in Thailand: a clinico-pathological correlation. Immunol Lett 25:199–206

Tayllor-Robinson A (1996) Nitric oxide in malaria: indicator of disease severity and infection control, Parasitol Today 12:208

Histopathological Diagnosis of Protozoan Infection Using Patients' Sera

Yutaka Tsutsumi

Summary. It is expected that the sera of patients suffering from infectious disease contain high-titer antibodies against the causative pathogens, particularly when the patients are not in an immunosuppressive state and host reactions such as abscess or granuloma are confirmed histologically. This chapter describes the utilization of diluted patients' sera as primary antibodies for the indirect immunoperoxidase identification of protozoan bodies in histopathological specimens routinely embedded in paraffin. Infectious agents such as *Entamoeba histolytica, Cryptosporidium parvum, Toxoplasma gondii, Leishmania major, Leishmania tropica,* and *Blastocystis hominis* were clearly demonstrable with an appreciable sensitivity and specificity. The method described here is simple, economic, useful, and beautiful in the histopathological diagnosis of protozoan infection and is also applicable to ultrastructural demonstration of the protozoan antigens.

Key Words: Immunoperoxidase method—Patient serum—Infectious disease—Paraffin section—Histopathological diagnosis—Cytological diagnosis—Immunoelectron microscopy—Protozoan infection—Amebic dysentery—Cryptosporidiosis—Toxoplasmosis—Cutaneous leishmaniosis—*Blastocystis hominis—Pneumocystis carinii*

Department of Pathology, Tokai University School of Medicine, Bohseidai, Isehara, Kanagawa 259-1193, Japan

Introduction

Of the 20 most common causes of death in the world, 16 are infectious diseases, 3 of which are protozoal disorders: malaria, amebic dysentery, and systemic leishmaniosis. Correct diagnosis of an infection leads patients directly to appropriate treatment and prophylaxis. The detection of pathogens in histopathology sections is required of pathologists. Immunohistochemical staining for pathogens is simple, specific, and sensitive. Actually, a wide variety of infectious agents have so far been detected immunohistochemically in routine histopathological and cytopathological specimens (Tsutsumi 1993). However, antibodies are not always available from commercial sources.

Specific high-titer antibodies can be expected to be readily detectable in the serum of the patient, particularly in the recovery stage of illness. The presence of tissue reactions such as abscess formation and granulomatous change indicates that the host immunocytes actively react to the pathogens in question. After 500- to 1000 fold dilution, the patient's serum can be applied as a convenient and economic primary antibody to formalin-fixed and paraffin-embedded sections. Indirect immunoperoxidase staining should be the choice of detection, because human endogenous IgG is only slightly demonstrated in tissue sections with this method (Tsutsumi 1994; Tsutsumi et al. 1991).

In this chapter, the author describes the sensitive demonstration of protozoan bodies in routinely processed paraffin sections, with the aid of the serum of those patients who were not in an immunosuppressive state. Examples include amebic dysentery, cryptosporidiosis, toxoplasmosis, cutaneous leishmaniosis, and *Blastocystis hominis* infection. The specificity is higher than expected, and the method is further applicable to localizing the protozoan antigens at the ultrastructural level.

Materials and Methods

Tissues obtained by biopsy, at surgery, or at autopsy were fixed routinely in 10% unbuffered formalin for a few days to 2 weeks. Specimens included the colon in amebic dysentery, the small intestine in cyptosporidiosis, the brain in toxoplasmosis, the skin in cutaneous leishmaniosis, cell blocks of cultured *Blastocystis hominis,* and the lung with *Pneumocystis carinii* infection. Ethanol-fixed sputum specimens of *P. carinii* pneumonia were also examined immunohistochemically. Infection of *Entamoeba histolytica*, *Cryptosporidium parvum*, *Toxoplasma gondii*, and *P. carinii* was seen in association with acquired immunodeficiency syndrome (AIDS) (Janoff and Smoth 1988; Pinching 1988).

The pathogens were visualized by the indirect immunoperoxidase technique in deparaffinized sections, as reported earlier (Tsutsumi 1994; Tsutsumi et al. 1991). The patients' sera, diluted at 1:500 to 1:1000, were incubated for 30 min. The presence of high-titer IgG antibody was confirmed fundamentally by immunofluorescence techniques in the respective patients' sera employed. Sera from AIDS patients were not utilized. Endogenous peroxidase activity was inhibited in methanol containing 0.3% hydrogen peroxide for 20 min. After diaminobenzidine reaction, the nuclei were counterstained with 5% methyl green. A mouse monoclonal antibody, EHK153, against *E. histolytica*, kindly supplied by Dr. Hiroshi Tachibana (Department of Parasitology, Tokai University School of Medicine, Isehara), was also used (Tachibana et al. 1990). For the identification of *P. carinii*, a commercial mouse monoclonal antibody, 3F6, from DAKO (Kyoto, Japan) was employed.

For ultrastructural localization of the antigens in frozen sections of buffered 4% paraformaldehyde-fixed pellets of cultured *B. hominis* established from nondiarrheal feces (Ziertdt 1991), the standard inverted beam capsule method for pre-embedding immunoelectron microscopy was performed (Hori et al. 1995).

Results

Protozoan pathogens were clearly identified at the site of infection in paraffin sections by employing diluted patient sera as primary antibodies in the indirect immunoperoxidase sequence. Presented here are microscopic and immunoperoxidase features of amebic dysentery (Fig. 1), cryptosporidiosis (Fig. 2), toxoplasmosis (Figs. 3, 4), African cutaneous leishmaniasis (Fig. 5), and cultured *B. hominis* (Fig. 6). In formalin-fixed, paraffin-embedded sections, endogenous human IgG was only meagerly demonstrated by the peroxidase-labeled secondary antibody (DAKO).

The trophozoites of *E. histolytica* were clearly demonstrated by high-titer patient serum without any background staining (Fig. 1, center). The

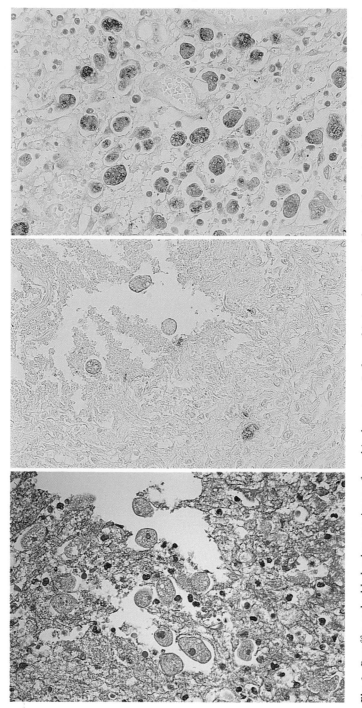

Fig. 1. Paraffin-embedded colon specimen of amebic dysentery. *Left*: amebic trophozoites with a single eosinophilic nucleus are seen at the ulcer base (H-E). *Center*: high-titer patient's serum detects the trophozoites (indirect immunoperoxidase). *Right*: monoclonal antibody EHK153 is strongly reactive in invasive protozoa in the colonic wall (indirect immunoperoxidase). ×100

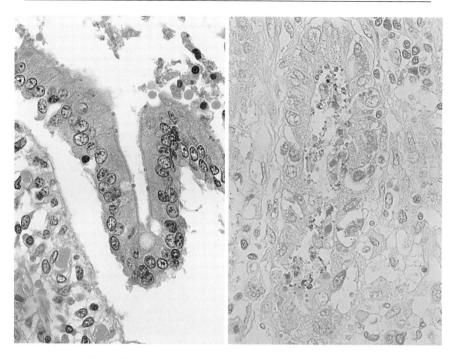

Fig. 2. Paraffin-embedded small bowel specimen in AIDS-associated cryptosporidiosis. *Left*: a few small amphophilic coccidioids along the brush border of the columnar cells are shown (H-E). *Right*: high-titer patient's serum is clearly reactive in the small protozoan bodies distributed on the luminal surface (indirect immunoperoxidase). ×200

invasive parasites were also strongly immunoreactive with the monoclonal antibody (Fig. 1, right).

Cryptosporidium parvum infection was clearly shown in the AIDS-associated enteropathic specimen by using the high-titer serum of an immunocompetent patient suffering from endemic protozoan diarrhea (Fig. 2).

The ruptured protozoan cysts in paraffin sections of AIDS-associated cerebral toxoplasmosis were immunoreactive with high-titer patient serum (Fig. 3). In a case of purulent meningitis associated with progressive supranuclear palsy, a few trophozoites of *T. gondii* were incidentally and unexpectedly identified in the meningeal space, confirming the diagnosis of *Toxoplasma* meningitis (Fig. 4). Intracerebral infection was also focally observed with this method.

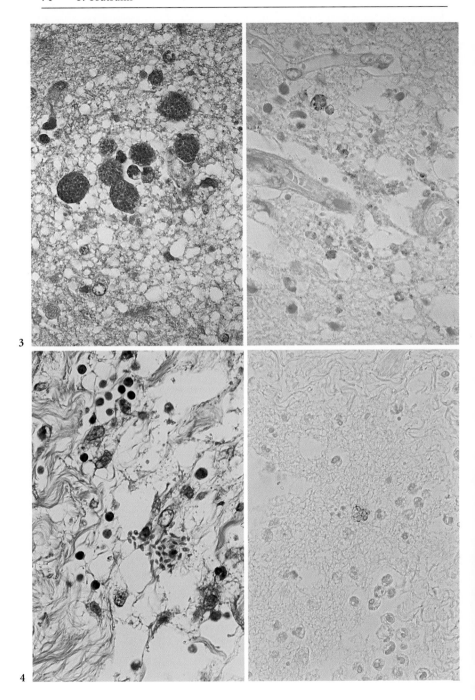

It is of note that the amastigotes (intracellular form) of *Leishmania major* in African-type cutaneous leishmaniosis were immunolabeled by the high-titer serum of a patient suffering from African-type skin disease (Fig. 5), but not by the serum of a patient with Indian-type disease caused by infection by *Leishmania tropica*.

The *B. hominis* antigens immunoreacted by high-titer patient serum (Fig. 6) were ultrastructurally localized by preembedding immunoelectron microscopy. As shown in Fig. 7, the plasma membranes were decorated by the patient's serum.

In paraffin sections of *P. carinii* pneumonia, the parasites (cysts) were clearly identified by the mouse monoclonal antibody. Immunoperoxidase identification was also possible in the ethanol-fixed sputum cytology specimen (Fig. 8).

Fig. 3. Paraffin-embedded brain specimen in AIDS-associated toxoplasmosis. *Left*: clusters of *Toxoplasma* cysts in the edematous cerebral tissues (H-E). *Right*: high-titer patient's serum identifies trophozoites dispersed from ruptured cysts in the brain (indirect immunoperoxidase). ×200

Fig. 4. *Toxoplasma gondii* trophozoites were unexpectedly identified in the meningeal space in paraffin sections of purulent meningitis. *Left*: a cluster of crescent-shaped trophozoites is seen in association with inflammatory infiltration (H-E). *Right*: *Toxoplasma* protozoan bodies in the meninges are visible as specific brown immunosignal (indirect immunoperoxidase). ×200

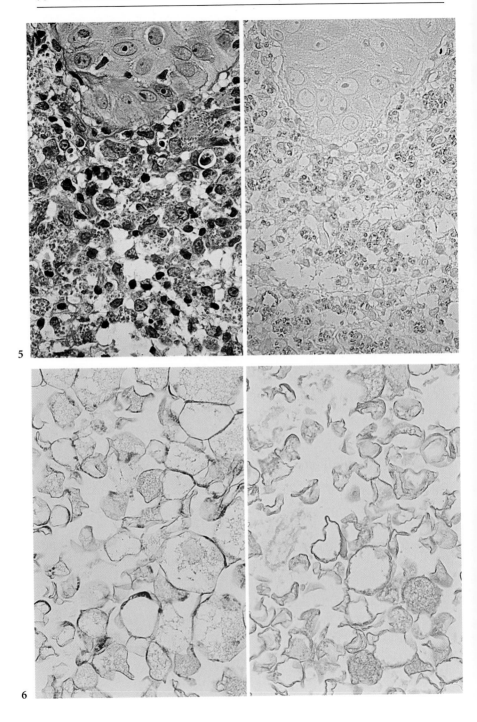

Fig. 5. Paraffin-embedded skin biopsy specimen in African cutaneous leishmaniosis caused by sandfly-mediated infection of *Leishmania major*. The dermis is densely infiltrated by macrophages, in which numerous phagocytized leishmanian bodies are clearly identified with the aid of the high-titer patient serum. The infectious agents were not labeled by the serum of a patient with *L. tropica infection*. *Left*, H-E; *right*, indirect immunoperoxidase. ×200

Fig. 6. Paraffin-embedded cytospun pellet of cultured *Blastocystis hominis*. *Left*: cystic organisms of large but varying size are grown in a monomorphous fashion (H-E). *Right*: high-titer patient's serum predominantly decorates the cell membranes of the pathogens (indirect immunoperoxidase). ×200

◀————————————————————————————————

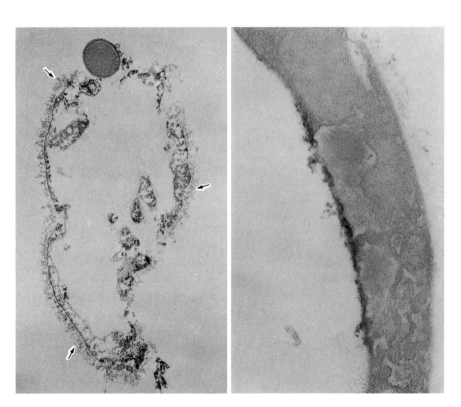

Fig. 7. Pre-embedding immunoelectron microscopic identification of *Blastocystis hominis* antigens in a prefixed pellet of cultured pathogens using patient's serum. *Left*: low-power view shows a membrane-associated positive reaction. Amorphous capsule-like substance around the cell body (*arrows*) is not reactive. ×5000 *Right*: high-power view exhibits positive signals in the inner membrane of the cystic structure. ×15 000

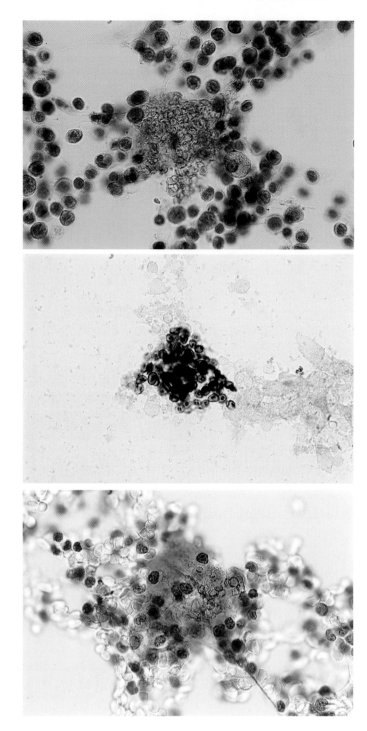

Fig. 8. Ethanol-fixed sputum cytology specimens containing *Pneumocystis carinii* in an AIDS patient. *Left*: a cluster of ghost red cell-like substance is seen by Papanicolaou staining. *Center*: Grocott-reactive *P. carinii* bodies (cysts) are clustered. *Right*: The monoclonal antibody 3F6 clearly identifies the clustered parasites (cysts) without any background staining (indirect immunoperoxidase with hematoxylin counterstaining). ×200

Discussion

Specific detection of infectious agents within the lesion undoubtedly is the key step for the histopathological diagnosis of infectious disease. Immunohistochemical demonstration of the pathogen seems to be a sensitive and practical approach. As described here, the trophozoites of *T. gondii* were incidentally but clearly demonstrated in paraffin sections in a case of purulent meningitis. When the cross-reactivity of the antibody is known, the result is beneficial for the patient, directly leading to the appropriate diagnosis, treatment, or prevention of outbreaks. For this purpose, the patients' sera can work as a potent and convenient weapon. The pathologist is requested to make a brief phone call to the clinician or clinical laboratory technician asking them to save a small aliquot of the target serum, after microscopically confirming the host response in histopathology specimens. This method is particularly effective when specific antibodies are not listed in a commercial catalog.

The indirect immunoperoxidase method should be the method of choice: techniques with high detectability, such as the streptavidin-biotinylated peroxidase complex method and labeled streptavidin-biotin method, expectedly result in background staining caused by the detection of endogenous IgG in tissue fluid (Tsutsumi 1993; Tsutsumi et al. 1991).

The specificity of immunostaining using patients' sera seems to be higher than expected, as described earlier (Tsutsumi et al. 1991). In fact, *L. major*, which causes African-type cutaneous leishmaniosis, could be differentiated from *L. tropica*, causing the Indian form. This implies that immunostaining with the patient's serum may distinguish even the subspecies of the pathogens seen in paraffin sections. Further detailed evaluations are needed for this applicability.

It is very important that the use of sera of patients with AIDS and of carriers of hepatitis B or C virus be avoided from the standpoint of biohazard and biosafety (Tsutsumi 1993; Tsutsumi et al. 1991). Moreover, protozoan diseases in AIDS commonly occur secondarily in a form of opportunistic infection (Janoff and Smoth 1988; Pinching 1988), strongly suggesting that the antibody titer against the pathogens is not elevated. In the case of *P. carinii* pneumonia, a typical opportunistic infection in AIDS, the commercially available monoclonal antibody worked very well. In the cytology specimen (Fig. 8), monoclonal antibodies are much better than patients' sera, because in the latter case, the secondary anti-human

IgG antibody detects body fluid IgG in the alcohol-treated specimen, resulting in high background staining.

Similarly, application of this technique to immunoelectron microscopic study using prefixed frozen sections would have some limitations because of the expected high background staining. In this study, frozen sections of pellets of cultured *B. hominis* were used for ultrastructural localization. The unfavorable effect by human IgG could be excluded under the condition employed.

In conclusion, the method described here is simple, economic, useful, and beautiful in the histopathological diagnosis of protozoan infection.

Acknowledgments. The author is deeply indebted to skillful technical assistance in the immunoperoxidase study by Kenji Kawai, M.T., and Akihiko Serizawa, M.T., Division of Diagnostic Pathology, Tokai University Hospital, Isehara. Valuable advice and suggestions, as well as the kind supply of patients' sera and monoclonal antibodies to *Entamoeba histolytica* and of cultured *Blastocystis hominis* by Kouichi Nagakura, Ph.D., Hiroshi Tachibana, Ph.D., and Prof. Yoshimasa Kaneda, M.D., Department of Parasitology, Tokai University School of Medicine, Isehara, are also cordially acknowledged. The intestinal specimen of cryptosporidiosis in AIDS and the high-titer serum of a patient with endemic *Cryptosporidium parvum* infection were kindly provided by Morio Koike, M.D., Department of Pathology, Tokyo Metropolitan Komagome Hospital, Tokyo, and Toshiro Kuroki, Ph.D., Kanagawa Hygienic Institute, Yokohama, Japan, respectively.

References

Hori S, Itoh H, Tsutsumi Y, Osamura RY (1995) Immunoelectron microscopic detection of chlamydial antigens in Papanicolaou-stained vaginal smears. Acta Cytol 39:835–837

Janoff EN, Smoth PD (1988) Perspectives on gastrointestinal infections in AIDS. Gastroenterol Clin North Am 17:451–463

Pinching AJ (1988) Factors affecting the natural history of human immunodeficiency virus infection. Immunodefic Rev 1:23–38

Tachibana H, Kobayashi S, Kato Y, Nagakura K, Kaneda Y, Takeuchi T (1990) Identification of a pathogenic isolate-specific 30,000-Mr antigen of *Entamoeba histolytica* by using a monoclonal antibody. Infect Immun 58:955–960

Tsutsumi Y (1993) Immunohistochemistry in infectious diseases (in Japanese). Byori-to-Rinsho 11:320–327

Tsutsumi Y (1994) Application of the immunoperoxidase method for histopathologic diagnosis of infectious diseases. Acta Histochem Cytochem 27:547–560

Tsutsumi Y, Nagakura K, Kawai K (1991) Use of patients' sera for immunoperoxidase demonstration of infectious agents in paraffin sections. Acta Pathol Jpn 41:673–679

Ziertdt CH (1991) *Blastocystis hominis.* Past and future. Clin Microbiol Rev 4:61–79

Molecular Genetics in Anisakid Nematodes from the Pacific Boreal Region

L. Paggi[1], S. Mattiucci[1], H. Ishikura[2], K. Kikuchi[2], N. Sato[2],
G. Nascetti[3], R. Cianchi[4], and L. Bullini[4]

Summary. Molecular studies were carried out on anisakid nematodes from the Pacific Boreal region, causal agents of human anisakiosis. Genetic markers showed that the three taxa detected in this area at the morphological level include at least six reproductively isolated biological species: *Anisakis simplex* sensu stricto and *A. simplex* C, belonging to the *A. simplex* complex; *Contracaecum osculatum* A, belonging to the *C. osculatum* complex; and *Pseudoterranova decipiens* B, *P. bulbosa*, and *P. azarasi*, belonging to the *P. decipiens* complex. Molecular keys for their routine identification are provided. Genetic relationships among members of the *A. simplex*, *C. osculatum*, and *P. decipiens* complexes are given by unweighted pair group cluster analysis (UPGMA) and multidimensional scaling ordination (MDS). Intermediate/paratenic fish hosts and definitive marine mammal hosts recorded for the considered species are provided: these are benthic-benthopelagic for *A. simplex* s. s. and *C. osculatum* C, and specialized benthic for *P. bulbosa* and *P. azarasi*. Maps are given showing collecting locations and geographic range of the species studied.

Key Words: Anisakid nematodes—*Anisakis simplex* sensu stricto—*Anisakis simplex* C—*Contracaecum osculatum* A—*Pseudoterranova decipiens* B—*Pseudoterranova bulbosa*—*Pseudoterranova azarasi*—

[1] Institute of Parasitology, University of Rome "La Sapienza," Piazzale Aldo Moro 5, I-00185 Rome, Italy
[2] Department of Pathology, Sapporo Medical University School of Medicine, Minami 1, Nishi 17, Chuo-ku, Sapporo 060-8556, Japan
[3] Department of Environmental Sciences, Tuscia University, Via S. C. De Lellis, I-01100 Viterbo, Italy
[4] Department of Genetics and Molecular Biology, University of Rome "La Sapienza," Via Lancisi 29, I-00161 Rome, Italy

Pacific   Boreal   region—Allozyme   markers—Biological   species—
Reproductive isolation—Molecular diagnostic keys—Genetic relationships—Host preferences—Geographic range

Introduction

The morphospecies *Anisakis simplex*, *Contracaecum osculatum*, and
Pseudoterranova decipiens, considered until recently cosmopolitan
and generalist, were found to include several biological species with different geographic distributions, life histories, and host preferences
(Mattiucci et al. 1997; Nascetti et al. 1983, 1986, 1993; Orecchia et al. 1994;
Paggi et al. 1991). This resolution was achieved by the use of genetic
markers as operational species descriptors; this approach has shown that,
in various taxonomic groups of endoparasitic helminths, morphospecies
may include a number of morphologically very similar but genetically
and ecologically differentiated taxa (sibling species), reproductively isolated in the field, with lack of gene exchange in sympatric areas in spite of
occasional F_1 hybrids (e.g., Aho et al. 1992; Baverstock et al. 1985;
Beveridge et al. 1993, 1994; Bullini 1985; Buron et al. 1986; Chilton et al.
1993; Chilton and Smales 1996; Nadler 1987, 1990; Paggi and Bullini 1994;
Paggi et al. 1985; Renaud et al. 1983; Reversat et al. 1989).

The aims of this chapter are (1) to analyze, by allozyme markers,
anisakid population samples from the Pacific Boreal region in order to
assess the biological species present in this area; (2) to estimate the genetic divergence of these species from related congeneric species; (3) to
analyze patterns of genetic relatedness among conspecific populations of
different geographic origin; (4) to clarify the life cycle of the considered
species, with particular regard to their intermediate/paratenic and definitive hosts; and (6) to assess species patterns of geographic distribution.

Materials and Methods

About 650 anisakid specimens were recovered from seven intermediate/
paratenic fish host species and from six definitive marine mammal host
species from Hokkaido Island, Sakhalin Islands, Bering Sea, and Pacific
Canada. The collecting sites, host species, and numbers of anisakid specimens tested are summarized in Table 1. Samples collected in the field

were deep-frozen and forwarded to Rome, Italy, where they were kept at
−80°C (for procedures, see Nascetti et al. 1986).

At the morphological level, the anisakid samples recovered from the
Pacific Boreal region included (1) *Anisakis* type I larvae (sensu Berland
1961; Shiraki 1974), a larval type found to correspond genetically to *A.
simplex* sensu lato (Orecchia et al. 1986), and *A. simplex* s. l. adults; (2)
Contracaecum larvae and *C. osculatum* s. l. adults; (3) *Pseudoterranova*
larvae and *P. decipiens* s. l. adults.

Single specimens were crushed in distilled water. Standard horizontal
starch gel electrophoresis was performed at 5°C at 7–9 V/cm for 3–6 h,
according to the gene–enzyme system. The following enzymes were routinely studied: idditol dehydrogenase (IDDH), malate dehydrogenase
(MDH), isocitrate dehydrogenase (IDH), 6-phosphogluconate dehydrogenase (6PGDH), glyceraldehyde-3-phosphate dehydrogenase (GAPDH),

Table 1. Collection data on the samples of *Anisakis simplex* sensu lato, *Contracaecum
osculatum* s. l. and *Pseudoterranova decipiens* s. l. tested from the Pacific Boreal region

Life stage	Number of parasites tested	Host	Collecting location
Anisakis simplex s.l.			
Adult	56	*Pseudorca crassidens*	Strait of Georgia (Pacific Canada)
Adult	29	*Phocoena phocoena*	Strait of Georgia (Pacific Canada)
L_4	5	*Phoca vitulina richardsi*	Strait of Georgia (Pacific Canada)
L_3	10	*Clupea harengus*	Strait of Georgia (Pacific Canada)
L_3	21	*Onchorhynchus gorbusha*	Sakhalin Islands
L_3	6	*Onchorhynchus keta*	Sakhalin Islands
L_3	5	*Gadus morhua macrocephalus*	Gulf of Anadyr (Bering Sea)
L_3	9	*Theragra chalcogramma*	Vancouver Island (Pacific Canada)
L_3	5	*Theragra chalcogramma*	Gulf of Anadyr (Bering Sea)
L_3	80	*Theragra chalcogramma*	Iwanai (Hokkaido Island)
L_3	26	*Theragra chalcogramma*	Nemuro (Hokkaido Island)
L_3	17	*Hippoglossus hippoglossus*	Gulf of Anadyr (Bering Sea)

Table 1. *Continued*

Life stage	Number of parasites tested	Host	Collecting location
Contracaecum osculatum s.l.			
Adult	37	*Phoca vitulina richardsi*	Crofton Bay (Pacific Canada)
Adult	78	*Erignathus barbatus*	Otaru Bay (Hokkaido)
L_3	4	*Gadus morhua macrocephalus*	Gulf of Anadyr (Bering Sea)
L_3	10	*Theragra chalcogramma*	Iwanai (Hokkaido Island)
L_3	7	*Theragra chalcogramma*	Gulf of Anadyr (Bering Sea)
L_3	2	*Hippoglossus hippolossus*	Gulf of Anadyr (Bering Sea)
Pseudoterranova decipiens s.l.			
Adult	29	*Eumetopias jubatus*	Rishiri Island (Hokkaido Island)
Adult	15	*Eumetopias jubatus*	Otaru Bay (Hokkaido Island)
Adult	52	*Eumetopias jubatus*	Iwanai (Hokkaido Island)
Adult	3	*Zalophus californianus*	Crofton Bay (Pacific Canada)
Adult	15	*Phoca vitulina richardsi*	Crofton Bay (Pacific Canada)
Adult	38	*Erignathus barbatus*	Otaru Bay (Hokkaido Island)
L_3	17	*Gadus morhua macrocephalus*	Gulf of Anadyr (Bering Sea)
L_3	46	*Gadus morhua macrocephalus*	Iwanai (Hokkaido Island)
L_3	23	*Myoxocephalus quadricornis*	Gulf of Anadyr (Bering Sea)
L_3	8	*Hippoglossus hippoglossus*	Gulf of Anadyr (Bering Sea)

L, Larval stage.

NADH dehydrogenase (NADHDH), superoxide dismutase (SOD), nucleoside phosphorylase (NP), aspartate aminotransferase (AAT), adenylate kinase (ADK), colorimetric esterase (cEST), fluorescent esterase (fEST), acid phosphatase (ACPH), leucine aminopeptidase (LAP), peptidase B (PEP B), peptidase C (PEP C), mannose phosphate isomerase (MPI), glucose phosphate isomerase (GPI), and phosphoglucomutase (PGM). Nineteen to 24 enzyme loci were analyzed, according to the species complex (Table 2).

Isozymes were numbered in order of decreasing electrophoretic mobility from the most anodal, and allozymes were numerically labeled accord-

Table 2. The enzymes studied, listed with their code number, quaternary structure, encoding loci, electrophoretic migration (+, anodal; −, cathodal), buffer systems, and staining procedures, for the samples of the *Anisakis simplex* (ASI), *Contracaecum osculatum* (COS), and *Pseudoterranova decipiens* (PDE) complexes analyzed from the Pacific Boreal region

Enzyme/code number	Encoding loci	Migration			Buffer system[a]			Staining procedure/reference
		ASI	COS	PDE	ASI	COS	PDE	
Idditol dehydrogenase (1.1.1.1)	Iddh	+	−	+	3	3	3	Nascetti et al. (1986), designated as *Sdh*
Malate dehydrogenase (1.1.1.3)	Mdh-1	+/−	+	+	5	5	5	Nascetti et al. (1986)
	Mdh-2		+	+		5	5	Nascetti et al. (1986)
	Mdh-3		−	−		5	5	Nascetti et al. (1986)
	Mdh-4		−			5		Nascetti et al. (1986)
Isocitrate dehydrogenase (1.1.1.4)	Idh	+	+	+	3	3	3	Nascetti et al. (1986)
6-Phosphogluconate dehydrogenase (1.1.1.4)	6Pgdh	+	+	+	5	5	5	Nascetti et al. (1986)
Glyceraldehyde-3-phosphate dehydrogenase (1.2.1.1)	Gapdh	+	+		3	3		Nascetti et al. (1986)
NADH dehydrogenase (1.6.99)	NADHdh	+		+	4		4	Nascetti et al. (1986)
Superoxide dismutase (1.15.1.1)	Sod-1	+	+	+	3, 6	3, 4	3, 6	Nascetti et al. (1986)
	Sod-2	−	−	−	3, 6	3, 4	3, 6	Nascetti et al. (1986)
Nucleoside phosphorylase (2.4.2.1)	Np	+	+	+	4, 7	4, 7	4	Modified from Nascetti et al. (1986); staining solution: 0.05 M phosphate buffer, pH 7.5
Aspartate amino transferase (2.6.1.1)	Aat-2	+/−	+	+	3	3	3	Nascetti et al. (1986)
Adenilate kinase (2.7.4.3)	Adk-2	−	−	−	5, 3	5, 3	5, 3	Nascetti et al. (1986)
Colorimetric esterase (3.1.1)	cEst-1	+	+	+	4, 2	4	4	Nascetti et al. (1986)
	cEst-2	+	+	+	4, 2	4	4	Nascetti et al. (1986)

Table 2. *Continued*

Enzyme/code number	Encoding loci	Migration			Buffer system[a]			Staining procedure/reference
		ASI	COS	PDE	ASI	COS	PDE	
Fluorescent esterase (3.1.1)	fEst-1		+			4, 7		Same as for carbonic anhydrase in Nascetti et al. (1986)
	fEst-2	+	+		7	4, 7		Nascetti et al. (1986)
Acid phosphatase (3.1.3.2)	Acph-2	−			2			Nascetti et al. (1986)
Leucine aminopeptidase (3.4.11)	Lap-1	+			2			Nascetti et al. (1986)
	Lap-2	+			2			Nascetti et al. (1986)
Peptidase (Leu-Leu) (3.4.11)	PepB	+			3			10 mg L-leucyl leucine, 3 mg peroxidase, 0.05 mg L-amino acid oxidase, 10 mg orthodianisidine, agar 0.8% in 30 ml Tris/HCl, 0.05 M pH 8
Peptidase (Leu-Ala) (3.4.11)	PepC-1	+	+	+	3	3	3	20 mg L-leucyl alanine, 3 mg peroxidase, 0.05 mg L-amino acid oxidase, 10 mg orthodianisidine, 10 mg MnC12, agar 0.8% in 30 ml Tris/HCl, 0.05 M pH 8
	PepC-2	+	+	+	3	3	3	
	PepC-3		+		3	3		
Mannose phosphate isomerase (5.3.1.8)	Mpi	+	+	+	4	4	4	Nascetti et al. (1986)
Glucose phosphate isomerase (5.3.1.9)	Gpi	+	+	+	4	4	4	Nascetti et al. (1986)
Phosphoglucomutase (5.4.2.2)	Pgm-1	+	+	+	7	6	6	Nascetti et al. (1986)
	Pgm-2	−	+		7	6	6	Nascetti et al. (1986)

[a] Buffer systems: 1, discontinuous Tris/citrate (Na), Poulik (1957); 2, discontinuous Tris/citrate (Li), modified from Poulik (1957); 3, continuous Tris/citrate, Selander et al. (1971); 4, Tris/versene/borate, Brewer and Sing (1970); 5, phosphate citrate, Harris (1966); 6, Tris-maleate, modified from Brewer and Sing (1970); 7, 0.1 M Tris-maleate, pH 7.8, Richardson et al. (1986).

ing to their mobility relative to the most common allele ($=100$) in reference populations of, respectively: (i) *A. pegreffii* from the Mediterranean Sea for the *A. simplex* complex (Nascetti et al. 1986); (ii) *C. osculatum* A from Hopen Island, Barents Sea, for the *C. osculatum* complex (Nascetti et al. 1993); and (iii) *P. decipiens* A from the Norwegian Sea for the *P. decipiens* complex (Paggi et al. 1991). The genetic structure of the Pacific Boreal samples was compared to populations previously studied for the three species complexes from different geographic areas.

The statistical significance of departures from Hardy–Weinberg equilibrium was estimated using both the chi-square test (χ^2) and *F* statistics (Wright 1943, 1951). χ^2 and *G* heterogeneity tests were performed to detect significant differences in allele frequencies among samples (Sokal and Rohlf 1981).

Genetic divergence of populations and species was estimated using the formulae proposed by Nei (1972) (standard genetic distance, D_{Nei}) and Rogers (1972), as modified by Wright (1978) (genetic distance, D_T). Unweighted pair group cluster analysis (UPGMA) from Nei's *D* values was carried out to show genetic relationships among populations, as well as a multidimensional scaling ordination (MDS) done from Rogers' D_T values with the Guttman (1968) method. BIOSYS software (Swofford and Selander 1989) was used for population analysis and SYSTAT (Wilkinson and Leland 1989) for multivariate analysis.

Results and Discussion

Anisakid Biological Species Detected in the Pacific Boreal Region

Genetic analysis by allozyme markers of larval and adult anisakid specimens recovered from Hokkaido Island, Sakhalin Island, the Bering Sea, and Pacific Canada has shown that at least six species are present in these areas: two belonging to the *Anisakis simplex* complex, genetically identified as *A. simplex* s. s. and *A. simplex* C; one belonging to the *Contracaecum osculatum* complex, identified as *C. osculatum* A; and three belonging to the *Pseudoterranova decipiens* complex, identified as *P. decipiens* B, *P. bulbosa*, and *P. azarasi*. On a morphological basis, only three species were recognized (*A. simplex* s. l., *P. decipiens* s. l., and *C. osculatum* s. l.). Three of the Pacific species detected genetically (*A. simplex* s. s., *A. simplex* C, and *C. osculatum* A) are sibling species, morphologically not distinguishable thus far from the other members of the respective complexes; *P. bulbosa* and *P. azarasi* were recently raised from synonymy with *P. decipiens* on the basis of a morphometric analysis of male tails carried out on material previously identified genetically (Mattiucci et al., in press); as for *P. decipiens* B, some morphometric differences from the other members of the complex were found by Paggi et al. (1991) and Di Deco et al. (1994).

Examples of molecular keys for species identification of the members of the *A. simplex*, *C. osculatum*, and *P. decipiens* complexes are given in Tables 3 through 5, respectively. These keys are based on a minimum number of loci and can be applied for routine tests of large anisakid

Table 3. Three examples of molecular (allozyme) keys for the identification of the members of the *Anisakis simplex* complex

		Locus	Alleles		Species
A	1.	*Mdh-1*	80, 90	→	*A. simplex* C
			100	→	2
	2.	*Adk-2*	100	→	*A. pegreffii*
			105	→	*A. simplex* sensu stricto
B		*PepC-1*	90	→	*A. simplex* s.s.
			100	→	*A. pegreffii*
			92	→	*A. simplex* C
C	1.	*PepC-2*	100	→	*A. pegreffii*
			96	→	2
	2.	*Adk-2*	100	→	*A. simplex* C
			105	→	*A. simplex* s.s.

Alleles with frequencies less than 0.05 were not included.
Data from Nascetti et al. (1986) and Mattiucci et al. (1997).

Table 4. An example of a molecular (allozyme) key for identification of members of the *Contracaecum osculatum* complex

	Locus	Alleles		Species
1.	*Mdh-3*	100	→	2
		110	→	*C. osculatum* C
2.	*Mdh-4*	100	→	3
		105	→	*C. osculatum* D
3.	*Adk-2*	100	→	4
		108	→	*C. osculatum* B
4.	*Sod-1*	100	→	*C. osculatum* A
		130, 125	→	*C. osculatum* E

Data from Nascetti et al. (1993) and Orecchia et al. (1994).

Table 5. Two examples of molecular (allozyme) keys for identification of the members of the *Pseudoterranova decipiens* complex

		Locus	Alleles		Species
A		*Pgm-1*	*100*	→	*P. decipiens* A
			103, 98	→	*P. bulbosa*
			105	→	*P. azarasi*
			107, 114	→	*P. decipiens* B
B	1	*Adk-2*	*100*	→	2
			107	→	*P. bulbosa*
	2	*Mdh-1*	*100*	→	*P. decipiens* A
			88, 98, 100	→	3
	3	*Aat-2*	*88, 103*	→	*P. decipiens* B
			92, 100	→	*P. decipiens* D

Alleles with frequencies less than 0.05 were not included.
Data from Paggi et al. (1991) and Mattiucci et al. (in press).

samples, allowing assignment of each specimen, at either the larval or adult stage, male or female, to the appropriate biological species.

Genetic and Evolutionary Relationships of the Pacific Boreal Anisakid Species

The genetic variation of anisakid samples from the Pacific Boreal region was compared to that of the members of the respective complexes from other geographic areas. Average genetic distance values within and among species of the three species complexes are given in Tables 6

Table 6. Average values and ranges (in parentheses) of genetic distance between members of the *Anisakis simplex* complex

	A. simplex s. s.	*A. simplex* C	*A. pegreffii*
A simplex s.s.	*0.018*	0.495	0.532
	(0.003–0.038)	(0.480–0.514)	(0.493–0.564)
A. simplex C	0.361	*0.046*	0.552
	(0.330–0.390)	*(0.004–0.088)*	(0.538–0.570)
A. pegreffii	0.399	0.453	*0.003*
	(0.334–0.445)	(0.419–0.492)	*(0.002–0.004)*

Values were calculated with the formulae by Nei (1972), below the diagonal, and by Rogers (1972) modified by Wright (1978), above the diagonal. Nei's genetic distance values found within the taxa are given along the diagonal.

Table 7. Average values and ranges (in parentheses) of genetic distance between members of the *Contracaecum osculatum* complex

	C. osculatum A	C. osculatum B	C. osculatum C	C. osculatum D	C. osculatum E
C. osculatum A	*0.009* *(0.002–0.017)*	0.574 (0.549–0.610)	0.640 (0.625–0.662)	0.477 (0.455–0.499)	0.412 (0.395–0.445)
C. osculatum B	0.500 (0.457–0.552)	*0.005* *(0.003–0.009)*	0.669 (0.661–0.676)	0.524 (0.511–0.536)	0.529 (0.523–0.535)
C. osculatum C	0.648 (0.623–0.669)	0.751 (0.735–0.772)	*0.002* *(0.002–0.002)*	0.638 (0.632–0.645)	0.597 (0.592–0.602)
C. osculatum D	0.322 (0.295–0.345)	0.413 (0.391–0.430)	0.670 (0.655–0.686)	*0.003* *(0.003–0.003)*	0.457 (0.450–0.464)
C. osculatum E	0.240 (0.222–0.268)	0.446 (0.438–0.455)	0.589 (0.578–0.600)	0.319 (0.308–0.331)	*0.001* *(0.001–0.001)*

Values were calculated with the formulae by Nei (1972), below the diagonal, and Rogers (1972), modified by Wright (1978), above the diagonal. Nei's genetic distance values found within taxa are given along the diagonal.

Table 8. Average values and ranges (in parentheses) of genetic distance between members of the *Pseudoterranova decipiens* complex

	P. decipiens A	P. decipiens B	P. bulbosa	P. azarasi
P. decipiens A	*0.005*	0.569	0.756	0.616
	(0.001–0.011)	(0.535–0.585)	(0.736–0.767)	(0.602–0.632)
P. decipiens B	0.518	*0.011*	0.665	0.531
	(0.387–0.967)	(0.001–0.023)	(0.654–0.674)	(0.504–0.546)
P. bulbosa	0.932	0.605	*0.004*	0.646
	(0.880–0.977)	(0.614–0.677)	(0.002–0.009)	(0.624–0.666)
P. azarasi	0.563	0.384	0.642	*0.021*
	(0.537–0.584)	(0.372–0.404)	(0.613–0.661)	(0.012–0.027)

Values were calculated with the formulae by Nei (1972), below the diagonal, and Rogers (1972), modified by Wright (1978), above the diagonal. Nei's genetic distance values found within taxa are given along the diagonal.

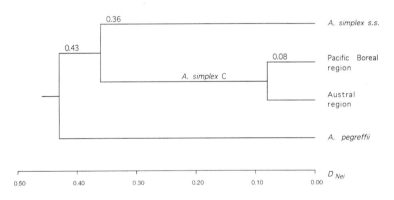

Fig. 1. UPGMA dendrogram calculated from Nei's values of genetic distance (D_{Nei}) shows the genetic relationships among members of the *Anisakis simplex* complex

through 8; genetic relationships among populations and species are summarized by the UPGMA dendrograms in Figs. 1 through 3 and by the plots of the first two dimensions of the MDS ordination analysis in Figs. 4 through 6.

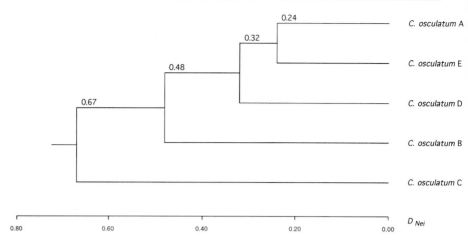

Fig. 2. UPGMA dendrogram calculated from Nei's values of genetic distance (D_{Nei}) shows the genetic relationships among members of the *Contracaecum osculatum* complex

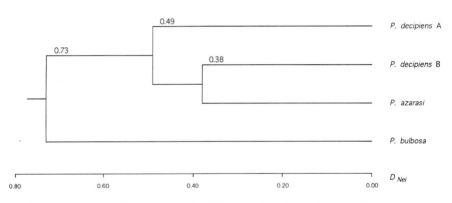

Fig. 3. UPGMA dendrogram calculated from Nei's values of genetic distance (D_{Nei}) shows the genetic relationships among members of the *Pseudoterranova decipiens* complex

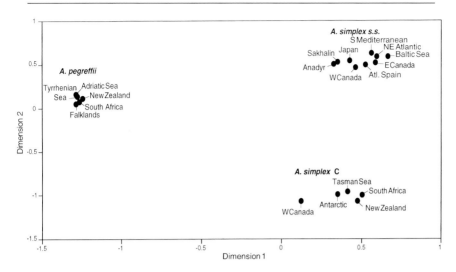

Fig. 4. Plot of the first two dimensions of a multidimensional scaling (MDS) analysis, obtained from Rogers' values of genetic distances (D_T), shows the genetic relationships among populations and species of the *Anisakis simplex* complex

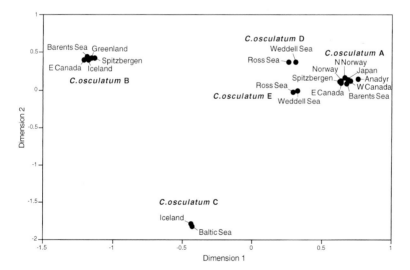

Fig. 5. Plot of the first two dimensions of a MDS analysis, obtained from Rogers' values of genetic distances (D_T), shows the genetic relationships among populations and species of the *Contracaecum osculatum* complex

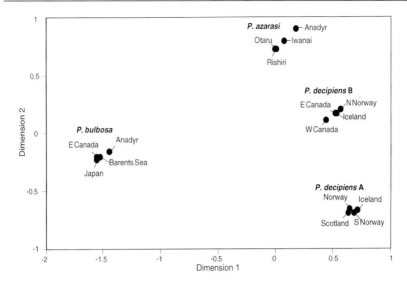

Fig. 6. Plot of the first two dimensions of a MDS ordination, obtained from Rogers' values of genetic distances (D_T), showing the genetic relationships among populations and species of the *Pseudoterranova decipiens* complex

Anisakis simplex *complex*

The genetic divergence between the two *Anisakis* species found in the Pacific Boreal region, *A. simplex* s. s and *A. simplex* C, is $D_{Nei} = 0.36$; both show a slightly higher genetic distance from the third member of the complex, *A. pegreffii* (Nascetti et al. 1986), with $D_{Nei} = 0.40$ and 0.45, respectively (see Table 6 and Fig. 1).

At the intraspecific level, the values of D_{Nei} found between populations of *A. simplex* s. s. ranged from 0.003 to 0.038; such a pattern of genetic distance is related to that of geographic distance (isolation by distance); average D_{Nei} values are 0.007 among Atlantic populations, 0.015 among Pacific ones, and 0.025 between the two groups. The highest value ($D_{Nei} = 0.038$) was found between the most distant populations, from the Baltic Sea and Hokkaido Island, Japan (see Fig. 4).

A more consistent intraspecific genetic distance was found in *A. simplex* C between the population from Pacific Canada and those from the Austral region (South Africa, New Zealand, Tasman Sea, and Antarctica); $D_{Nei} = 0.085$. The taxonomic rank of these two population groups is still to be assessed (Mattiucci et al. 1997).

Contracaecum osculatum *complex*

Only one member of the *C. osculatum* complex, *C. osculatum* A, was detected in the Pacific Boreal region (Pacific Canada, Hokkaido Island, Bering Sea). This species is related more to the two Antarctic species, *C. osculatum* E (D_{Nei} = 0.24) and *C. osculatum* D (D_{Nei} = 0.32) than to the other Boreal members of the complex, *C. osculatum* B (D_{Nei} = 0.50) and *C. osculatum* C (D_{Nei} = 0.65) (Table 7 and Fig. 2). This indicates recent multiple events of colonization of the Antarctic region from a common ancestor (Arduino et al. 1995; Bullini et al. 1994; Orecchia et al. 1994). At the intraspecific level, the values of D_{Nei} within *C. osculatum* A ranged from 0.002 to 0.017, with an average of 0.009. Average D_{Nei} values are 0.004 within Northern Atlantic populations, 0.008 among Pacific populations, and 0.018 between the two groups, showing a geographic pattern of variation, although less marked than in *A. simplex* s. s. (Fig. 5).

Pseudoterranova decipiens *complex*

The three members of the *P. decipiens* complex found in the Pacific region showed the following values of genetic divergence: D_{Nei} = 0.38 between *P. azarasi* and *P. decipiens* B, D_{Nei} = 0.60 between *P. bulbosa* and *P. decipiens* B, and D_{Nei} = 0.64 between *P. azarasi* and *P. bulbosa* (Table 8 and Fig. 3). At the intraspecific level, the lowest genetic heterogeneity was found within *P. bulbosa*, in spite of geographic distances, with an average D_{Nei} = 0.004. The highest intraspecific differentiation was detected within *P. azarasi*; e.g., the sample from Anadyr (Bering Sea) showed a value of D_{Nei} = 0.026 from conspecific Japanese samples. Both *P. decipiens* B and *P. azarasi* showed a relationship between geographic and genetic distances, whereas higher levels of gene exchange were detected within *P. bulbosa* (see Fig. 6).

Life Cycle and Ecological Niche of Pacific Boreal Anisakid Species

The intermediate/paratenic and definitive hosts recorded in the Pacific region for the three anisakid species complexes *A. simplex* s. l., *C. osculatum* s. l., and *P. decipiens* s. l., respectively, are listed in Tables 9 through 11 and examined here.

Anisakis simplex *complex*

A. simplex C from Pacific Canada has been recovered so far only from the false killer whale, *Pseudorca crassidens*, together with *A. simplex* s. s. In the Austral region, adults were recovered in the long-finned pilot whale *Globicephala melaena* and larval specimens in the gadid fishes *Parapercis colias* and *Pseudophycis bachus*, the trachichthyid *Hoplostethus atlanticus*, and the gempylid *Thyrsites atun* (Mattiucci et al. 1997). *A. simplex* C was also collected in the southern elephant seal, *Mirounga leonina*, from the Antarctic. A greater number of hosts was recorded for *A. simplex* s. s. from the Pacific, with 2 marine mammal and 6 fish species (see Table 9). Among the latter, 3 species (*Onchorhynchus gorbusha*, *Onchorhynchus keta*, and *Hippoglossus hippoglossus*) were not listed in the previous review of *A. simplex* s.s. hosts (Mattiucci et al. 1997); accordingly, the number of host species of *A. simplex* so far recorded from all the world rises to 27, including 2 squid, 17 fish, and 8 marine mammals. The benthic-benthopelagic habitat of *A. simplex* s.s. hosts is confirmed by the new data.

Table 9. Definitive (marine mammals) and intermediate/paratenic (fish) hosts identified so far for members of the *Anisakis simplex* complex in the Pacific Boreal region

Host species	*A. simplex* s. s.	*A. simplex* C
Marine mammals		
Pseudorca crassidens	*	*
Phocoena phocoena	*	
Fish		
Clupea harengus	*	
Onchorhynchus gorbusha	*	
Onchorhynchus keta	*	
Gadus morhua macrocephalus	*	
Theragra chalcogramma	*	
Hippoglossus hippoglossus	*	

Table 10. Definitive (marine mammals) and intermediate/paratenic (fish) hosts identified so far for members of the *Contracaecum osculatum* complex in the Pacific Boreal region

Host species	*C. osculatum* A
Marine mammals	
Phoca vitulina richardsi	*
Erignathus barbatus	*
Fish	
Gadus morhua macrocephalus	*
Theragra chalcogramma	*
Hippoglossus hippoglossus	*

Contracaecum osculatum *complex*

The Pacific populations of *C. osculatum* A were recovered from two definitive host species, the bearded seal *Erignathus barbatus* and the Pacific harbor seal *Phoca vitulina richardsi* (see Table 10). The former, which has a northern boreal distribution, was found to be the main definitive host of *C. osculatum* A also in the Atlantic region (Nascetti et al. 1993), together with, to a lesser extent, the gray seal *Halichoerus grypus*, which is distributed in the North Atlantic and Baltic Sea. As to intermediate/paratenic hosts, three fish species were detected in this study: *Gadus morhua macrocephalus*, *Theragra chalcogramma*, and *Hippoglossus hippoglossus*. The hosts so far detected for *C. osculatum* A throughout its range are either benthic (*E. barbatus*, *H. hippoglossus*) or benthopelagic (*P. vitulina richardsi*, *H. grypus*, *G. morhua*, *T. chalcogramma*).

Pseudoterranova decipiens *complex*

The population of *P. decipiens* B from Pacific Canada was recovered from the California sea lion *Zalophus californianus* and the Pacific harbor seal *P. vitulina richardsi*, both distributed along the western American coast and benthopelagic (see Table 11). In the North Atlantic region, *P. decipiens* B was recovered mainly from the nominal subspecies of the harbor seal, *P. vitulina vitulina*, and from the gray seal, *Halichoerus grypus* (Paggi et al. 1991).

As to *P. bulbosa*, it was detected only in the bearded seal *Erignathus barbatus*, in the Pacific as well as in the Atlantic region. Its intermediate/

Table 11. Definitive (marine mammals) and intermediate/paratenic (fish) hosts identified so far for members of the *Pseudoterranova decipiens* complex in the Pacific Boreal region

Host species	*P. decipiens* B	*P. bulbosa*	*P. azarasi*
Marine mammals			
Eumetopias jubatus			*
Zalophus californianus	*		
Phoca vitulina richardsi	*		
Erignathus barbatus		*	*
Fish			
Gadus morhua macrocephalus		*	*
Myoxocephalus quadricornis		*	
Hippoglossus hippoglossus		*	*

paratenic hosts detected in the Pacific region are *Gadus morhua macrocephalus*, *Myoxocephalus quadricornis*, and *Hippoglossus hippoglossus*, whereas in the Atlantic region the flatfishes *Hippoglossoides platessoides* and *Reinhardtius hippoglossoides* (Paggi et al. 1991). The hosts so far detected for *P. bulbosa* are specialized benthic species, with the exception of *G. morhua*, which is benthopelagic.

Pseudoterranova azarasi was recovered in a mixed infection with *P. bulbosa* in a bearded seal from Hokkaido Island; it was also found in the steller sea lion, *Eumetopias jubatus*. As to its intermediate/paratenic hosts, they were also shared with *P. bulbosa*: *Gadus morhua macrocephalus* and *Hippoglossus hippoglossus*. These findings suggest a similar life cycle for *P. bulbosa* and *P. azarasi*, carried out in benthic species.

Patterns of Geographic Distribution

The maps in Figs. 7 through 9 summarize the collecting sites of the members so far detected of the *A. simplex*, *C. osculatum*, and *P. decipiens* complexes, respectively. Eight species of the three complexes were found in the Boreal temperate region, above 30°N; the other two, *A. simplex* C and *A. pegreffii*, have a Boreal-Austral range, while *C. osculatum* D and E are from Antarctica. Among the Boreal species, *A. simplex* s.s., *C. osculatum* A, *P. decipiens* B, and *P. bulbosa* are circum-Boreal; *C. osculatum* B, *C. osculatum* C, and *P. decipiens* A have been detected so far only in the Atlantic region; and *P. azarasi* has been found so far only in Pacific waters (Hokkaido Island and Bering Sea).

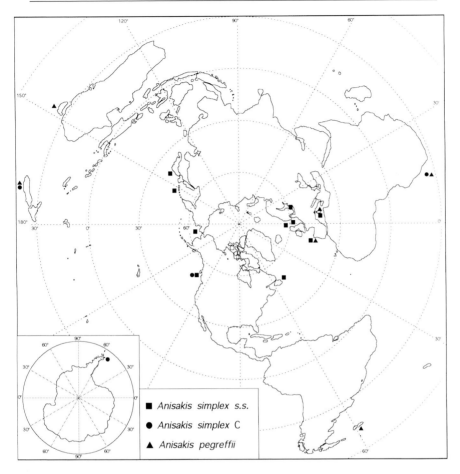

Fig. 7. Map of the collecting sites of members of the *Anisakis simplex* complex. Data are from Mattiucci et al. (1997) and the current study

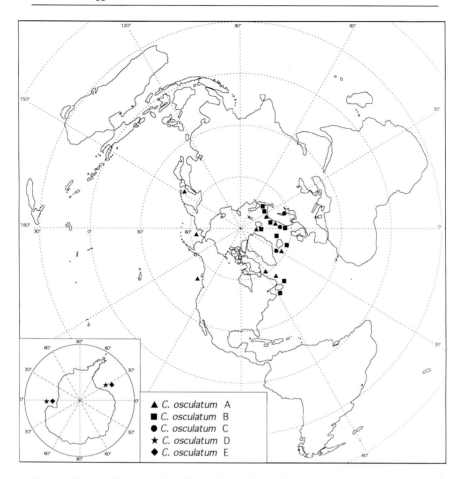

Fig. 8. Map of the collecting sites of members of the *Contracaecum osculatum* complex. Data are from Nascetti et al. (1993), Orecchia et al. (1994), and the current study

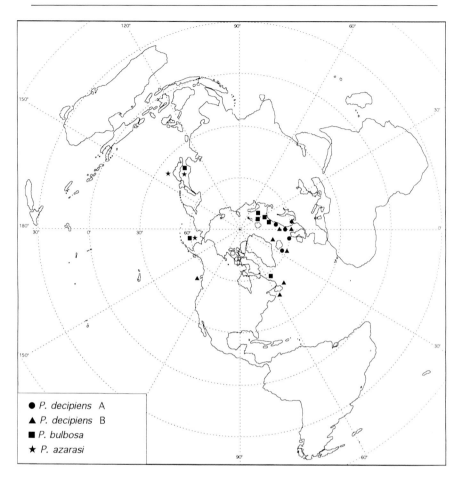

Fig. 9. Map of the collecting sites of members of the *Pseudoterranova decipiens* complex. Data are from Paggi et al. (1991), Mattiucci et al. (in press), and the current study

Concluding Remarks

This study is concerned with three anisakid species complexes, infecting marine mammals and fish, from the Pacific Boreal region. The study of these complexes by molecular markers allowed to detect different biological species, irrespective of their morphological differentiation, and to define their genetic variation, host preferences, and geographic distribution. All the anisakid species detected in the Pacific region are possibly involved as causal agents of human anisakiosis, which reaches significant peaks in this area. The study by molecular diagnostic keys of parasites surgically removed from patients will allow assessment of their relative epidemiological role.

Acknowledgments. We thank Dr. Dmitri G. Tseitlin (Russian Academy of Sciences, Moscow), for his valuable contribution in collecting samples from Sakhalin Islands and Anadyr, and Dr. Andrea Ungaro for drawing the figures. The research was supported by grants from Ministero delle Risorse Agricole, Alimentari e Forestali (Direzione Generale della Pesca), Italy.

References

Aho JM, Mulvey M, Jacobson K, Esch GW (1992) Genetic differentiation among congeneric acanthocephalans in the yellow-bellied slider turtle. J Parasitol 78:974–981

Arduino P, Nascetti G, Cianchi R, Plötz J, Mattiucci S, D'Amelio S, Paggi L, Orecchia P, Bullini L (1995) Isozyme variation and taxonomic rank of *Contracaecum radiatum* (v. Linstow, 1907) from the Antarctic Ocean (Nematoda, Ascaridoidea). Syst Parasitol 30:1–9

Baverstock PR, Adams M, Beveridge I (1985) Biochemical differentiation in bile duct cestodes and their marsupial hosts. Mol Biochem Evol 2:321–337

Berland B (1961) Nematodes from some Norwegian marine fishes. Sarsia 2:1–50

Beveridge I, Chilton NB, Andrews RH (1993) Sibling species within *Macropostrongyloides baylisi* (Nematoda: Strongyloidea) from macropodid marsupials detected by allozyme electrophoresis. Int J Parasitol 23:21–32

Beveridge I, Chilton NB, Andrews RH (1994) A morphological and electrophoretic study of *Rugopharynx zeta* (Johnston and Mawson, 1939) (Nematoda: Strongyloidea), with the description of a new species, *R. mawsonae*, from the black-striped wallaby, *Macropus dorsalis*. Syst Parasitol 27:159–171

Brewer GJ, Sing CF (1970) An introduction to isozyme techniques. Academic Press, New York

Bullini L (1985) The electrophoretic approach to the study of parasites and vectors. Parassitologia (Rome) 27:1–11

Bullini L, Arduino P, Cianchi R, Nascetti G, D'Amelio S, Mattiucci S, Paggi L, Orecchia P (1994) Genetic and ecological studies on nematode endoparasites of the genera *Contracaecum* and *Pseudoterranova* in the Antarctic and Arctic-Boreal regions. In: Battaglia B, Bisol PM, Varotto V (eds) Proceedings, 2nd meeting on Antarctic Biology, Padova 1992. Scienza e Cultura, Aldo Martello, Ed. Univ. Patav., Padova, Italy, pp 131–146

Buron de I, Renaud F, Euzet L (1986) Speciation and specificity of acanthocephalans. Genetic and morphological studies of *Acanthocephaloides geneticus* sp. nov. parasitizing *Arnoglossus laterna* (Bothidae) from the Mediterranean littoral (Sète-France). Parasitology 92:165–171

Chilton NB, Smales RL (1996) An electrophoretic and morphological analysis of *Labiostrongylus* (*Labiomultiplex*) *uncinatus* (Nematoda: Cloacinidae), with the description of a new species, *L. contiguus*, from *Macropus parryi* (Marsupialia: Macropodidae). Syst Parasitol 35:49–57

Chilton NB, Beveridge I, Andrew RH (1993) Electrophoretic comparison of *Rugopharynz longibursaris* Kung and *Rugopharynx omega* Beveridge (Nematoda: Strongyloidea), with the description of *R. sigma* n. sp. from the red-legegd pademelon. Syst Parasitol 26:159–169

Di Deco MA, Orecchia P, Paggi L, Petrarca V (1994) Morphometric stepwise discriminant analysis of three genetically identified species within *Pseudoterranova decipiens* (Krabbe, 1878) (Nematoda: Ascaridida). Syst Parasitol 29:81–88

Guttman LA (1968) A general nonmetric technique for finding the smallest coordinate space for a configuration of points. Psychometrica 33:469–506

Harris H (1966) Enzymes polymorphism in man. Proc R Soc Lond Ser B 164:298–310

Mattiucci S, Nascetti G, Cianchi R, Paggi L, Arduino P, Margolis L, Brattey J, Webb S, D'Amelio S, Orecchia P, Bullini L (1997) Genetic and ecological data on the *Anisakis simplex* complex, with evidence for a new species (Nematoda, Ascaridoidea, Anisakidae). J Parasitol 83:401–416

Mattiucci S, Paggi L, Nascetti G, Ishikura H, Kikuchi K, Sato N, Cianchi R, Bullini L (1998) Allozyme and morphological identification of *Anisakis*, *Contracaecum* and *Pseudoterranova* from Japanese waters (Nematoda, Ascaridoidea). Syst Parasitol (in press)

Nadler SA (1987) Biochemical and immunological systematics in some ascaridoid nematodes: genetic divergence between congeners. J Parasitol 73:811–816

Nadler SA (1990) Molecular approaches to studying helminth population genetics and phylogeny. Int J Parasitol 20:11–29

Nascetti G, Paggi L, Orecchia P, Mattiucci S, Bullini L (1983) Two sibling species within *Anisakis simplex* (Ascaridida: Anisakidae). Parassitologia (Rome) 25:239–241

Nascetti G, Paggi L, Orecchia P, Smith JW, Mattiucci S, Bullini L (1986) Electrophoretic studies on the *Anisakis simplex* complex (Ascaridida: Anisakidae) from the Mediterranean and North-East Atlantic. Int J Parasitol 16:633–640

Nascetti G, Cianchi R, Mattiucci S, D'Amelio S, Orecchia P, Paggi L, Brattey J, Berland B, Smith JW, Bullini L (1993) Three sibling species within *Contracaecum osculatum* (Nematoda, Ascaridida, Ascaridoidea) from the Atlantic Arctic-Boreal region: reproductive isolation and host preferences. Int J Parasitol 23:105–120

Nei M (1972) Genetic distance between populations. Am Nat 106:283–292

Orecchia P, Paggi L, Mattiucci S, Smith JW, Nascetti G, Bullini L (1986) Electrophoretic identification of larvae and adults of *Anisakis* (Ascaridida: Anisakidae). J Helminthol 60:331–339

Orecchia P, Mattiucci S, D'Amelio S, Paggi L, Plötz J, Cianchi R, Nascetti G, Arduino P, Bullini L (1994) Two new members in the *Contracaecum osculatum* complex (Nematoda, Ascaridoidea) from the Antarctic. Int J Parasitol 24:367–377

Paggi L, Bullini L (1994) Molecular taxonomy in anisakids. Bull Scand Soc Parasitol 4:25–39

Paggi L, Nascetti G, Orecchia P, Mattiucci S, Bullini L (1985) Biochemical taxonomy of ascaridoid nematodes. Parassitologia 27:105–112

Paggi L, Nascetti G, Cianchi R, Orecchia P, Mattiucci S, D'Amelio S, Berland B, Brattey J, Smith JW, Bullini L (1991) Genetic evidence for three species within *Pseudoterranova decipiens* (Nematoda, Ascaridida, Ascaridoidea) in the North Atlantic and Norwegian and Barents seas. Int J Parasitol 21:195–212

Poulik MD (1957) Starch gel electrophoresis in a discontinuous system of buffers. Nature (Lond) 180:1477

Renaud F, Gabrion C, Pasteur N (1983) Le complexe *Bothriocephalus scorpii* (Mueller, 1776): différenciations par électrophorèse enzymatique des espèces parasites du turbot (*Psetta maxima*) et de la barbue (*Scophthalmus rhombus*). C R Acad Sci Paris 296:127–129

Reversat J, Renaud F, Maillard C (1989) Biology of parasite populations: the differential specificity of the genus *Helicometra* Odhner, 1902 (Trematoda: Opecoelidae) in the Mediterranean Sea demonstrated by enzyme electrophoresis. Int J Parasitol 19:885–890

Richardson BJ, Baverstock PR, Adams M (1986) Allozyme electrophoresis. A handbook for animal systematics and population studies. Academic Press, Sydney, p 410

Rogers JS (1972) Measures of genetic similarities and genetic distance. Stud Genet VII Univ Texas Publ (Austin) 7213:145–153

Selander RK, Smith MH, Yang SY, Johnson WE, Gentry JB (1971) Biochemical polymorphism and systematics in the genus *Peromyscus*. Variation of the old-field mouse (*Peromyscus polionotus*). Stud Genet VI Univ Texas Publ (Austin) 7103:49–90

Shiraki T (1974) Larval nematodes of family Anisakidae (Nematoda) in the Northern Sea of Japan—as causative agent of eosinophilic phlegmone or granuloma in the human gastrointestinal tract. Acta Med Biol 22:57–98

Sokal RR, Rohlf FJ (1981) Biometry, 2nd edn. Freeman, New York, p 859

Swofford DL, Selander RB (1989) BIOSYS-1: a computer program for the analysis of allelic variation in population genetics and biochemical systematics. Release 1.7. Illinois Natural History Survey, p 31

Wilkinson L, Leland FJ (1989) SYSTAT: the system for statistics. SYSTAT, Evanson, Illinois, p 600

Wright S (1943) Isolation by distance. Genetics 28:114–138
Wright S (1951) The genetical structure of populations. Ann Eugen 15:323–354
Wright S (1978) Evolution and the genetics of populations. 4. Variability within and among natural populations. University of Chicago Press, Chicago, Illinois, p 580

Anisakidosis: Global Point of View

SHUJI TAKAHASHI, HAJIME ISHIKURA, and KOKICHI KIKUCHI

Summary. Anisakidosis, a human parasitic disease, is one of the zoonoses caused by certain types of anisakid nematodes. More than 30 000 cases have been reported in the world, and most of the cases have occurred in Japan because of the custom of eating raw fish that are the intermediate (paratenic) host. On Hokkaido Island in Japan, a relatively high incidence of anisakidosis is caused by *Pseudoterranova decipiens* as well as *Anisakis simplex*. It became apparent that *Pseudoterranova decipiens* was carried by Steller's sea lions (*Eumetopias jubata*) from their natural habitats, Komandor Island and Moneron Island of Sakhalin. According to these observations, we speculated that the incidence of anisakidosis and the infection patterns of the responsible worms depend on the distribution of the intermediate (paratenic) and final hosts of the anisakid worms, which is influenced by sea current and climate.

Key Words: Occurrence of anisakidosis—Epidemiology—Life cycle— Intermediate host—Final host

Introduction

Anisakidosis is a disease caused by anisakid larvae, having clinical manifestations such as abdominal pain and ileus after eating raw fish. Many anisakid species responsible for human anisakidosis have now been identified: *Anisakis simplex* (A.), *Pseudoterranova decipiens* (P.), *Contracaecum osculatum* (C.), *Hysterothylacium aduncum* (H.), and *Porrocaecum reticulatum*, which belongs to the family Ascarididae (Ishikura et al. 1993; Takahashi et al. 1986, 1990; Yagihashi et al. 1989).

Department of Pathology, Sapporo Medical University School of Medicine, Minami 1, Nishi 17, Chuo-ku, Sapporo 060-8556, Japan

In this study, "anisakidosis" means the disease caused by *Anisakis* and "*Anisakis*-related" species, and "anisakiosis" means the disease caused only by the *Anisakis* worm. Although anisakiosis is a very common disease among Japanese people, the factors affecting the pathogenesis and the incidence, the responsible nematodes, and the locale of anisakiosis with certain types of larvae remain to be elucidated.

We investigated the incidence, responsible nematodes, and location of anisakiosis in the world from references, with special reference to the concentration of anisakidosis by *Pseudoterranova decipiens* in Hokkaido, Japan. We propose that the distribution of the intermediate (paratenic) and final hosts may determine the locality and variation of anisakidosis.

Materials and Methods

Analysis of the Worldwide Incidence of Anisakidosis

We analyzed the incidence of anisakidosis throughout the world by collecting information from collaborating institutes in Japan and references from the medical database system (Medline, SilverPlatter International, USA), the CAB databank in the U.K., and by studying *Helminthological Abstracts*.

Analysis of Anisakid Nematodes in Marine Mammals

We obtained stomachs of *Theragra chalcogramma* for analysis of infection by anisakid species. These sea mammals were caught off the coast of Iwanai Fishery Port in Hokkaido (N 42°50′, E 140°25′) on January 25, 1986, or in Nemuro Strait between Hokkaido and Ostrov Knashr (N 43°0′, E 145°0′) on February 2, 1986. The anisakid and anisakid-related nematodes were identified by morphological investigation as reported in a previous publication.

Results and Discussion

Statistics of Global Incidence of Anisakidosis

Anisakidosis is defined as the disease caused by infection with Anisakidae worms including *Anisakis simplex, Pseudoterranova*

decipiens, Contracaecum osculatum, and *Hysterothylacium aduncum.*
Ascariosis, which is caused by infection with *Porrocaecum reticulatum*
(P.r.), resembles anisakidosis morphologically. Accordingly, it is important to identify the worm responsible for each type of anisakidosis. The
worms can be identified by their morphological features. For example,
A. simplex does not have a cecum, but *H. aduncum* has both intestinal
and gastric ceca and *P. decipiens* has an intestinal cecum. We can
also discriminate between the nematodes by their lips, lateral cords,
and tail. Most of the worms are larval forms, but human infection with
adult forms is also reported for certain types of Anisakidae, such as *P.
decipiens.*

There are subtle differences in the clinical symptoms among the worms
responsible. *A. simplex* frequently causes severe colic pain in gastric
anisakidosis, but *P. decipiens* seems to cause relatively mild clinical symptoms, probably because of the different preimmune status of humans. We
often meet difficulty in identification of the nematodes from the literature, mostly because of the lack of an adequate description and the ab-
sence of a stable classification method of the nematodes. Nevertheless, we
tried to analyze the incidence of anisakidosis worldwide and the worms
responsible by an investigation of the literature. To date, we have found
more than 30000 cases of anisakidosis in the literature (Table 1). As
expected, most of the cases were from Japan, because of the custom to
eating raw fish as sushi or sashimi. We believe that the number of reported cases in Japan is just the "tip of the iceberg," and we estimate that
the actual incidence of anisakidosis might be 5- to 10 fold greater in
Japan.

Although physicians are aware of gastric anisakidosis in Japan because
of its typical symptoms and because it can easily be diagnosed and treated
by endoscopy, intestinal anisakidosis on the other hand is difficult
to diagnose. We established a serodiagnostic kit for the intestinal
anisakidosis caused by *A. simplex* (Takahashi et al. 1986, 1990; Yagihashi
et al. 1989). Anisakidosis is recognized not only in Japan but also in many
other countries including Korea, Netherlands, and France (Ishikura et al.
1996a). Because of the recent popularity of healthy Japanese food,
anisakidosis seems to be increasing in developed Western countries such
as the United States. Since van Thiel reported the first case of anisakidosis
in the Netherlands, it has become mandatory to freeze fish before serving
them in that country.

Table 1. Occurrence of anisakidosis in the world

	Anisakis simplex		H.A.	Pseudoterranova		Contracaecum sp.	Hysterothylacum sp.	R.K.C.	Unknown	Total
	G.	I.		G.	I.					
Japan	26823	1057	142	805	1	2	1	1338	520	30689
Netherland	3	289	0	0	0	0	0	0	0	292
Korea	227	11	0	6	1	2	0	0	0	247
France	57	25	0	0	0	0	0	0	32	114
Germany	13	76	0	0	0	0	0	0	7	96
U.S.A.	25	31	0	12	2	0	0	0	2	72
U.K.	2	3	0	2	0	0	0	0	5	12
Belgium	0	9	0	0	0	0	0	0	0	9
Norway	0	1	0	0	0	0	0	0	5	6
Poland	0	0	0	0	0	0	0	0	5	5
Chile	1	0	0	1	0	0	0	0	3	5
Spain	1	3	0	1	0	0	0	0	1	6
Canada	2	0	0	2	0	0	0	0	0	4

Sweden	1	2	0	0	0	0	0	0	0	3
Brazil	0	0	0	0	0	0	0	0	2	2
Israel	2	0	0	0	0	0	0	0	0	2
Denmark	0	0	0	0	0	0	0	0	1	1
Italy	0	1	0	0	0	0	0	0	1	1
New Zealand	0	0	0	0	0	0	0	0	0	1
Greenland	0	0	0	1	0	0	0	0	0	1
Western Samo	0	0	0	0	0	0	0	0	1	1
Taiwan	0	0	0	0	0	0	0	0	1	1
Tahiti	1	0	0	0	0	0	0	0	0	1
Mexico	0	1	0	0	0	0	0	0	0	1
Finland	0	1	0	0	0	0	0	0	0	1
Thailand	0	1	0	0	0	0	0	0	0	1
Oman	1	0	0	0	0	0	1	0	0	1
Totals	27159	1511	142	830	4	4	1	1338	586	31575

H.A., heterogeneous anisakiosis; R.K.C., reagent kid component. Data through December 1996.

Anisakidosis from *Pseudoterranova decipiens* in Japan

Most anisakidosis is caused by *A. simplex*, but there are some reports of infection by other anisakid nematodes. In Japan, it is of note that a certain number of cases of anisakidosis are caused by *P. decipiens*. Further analysis has revealed that the anisakidosis caused by *P. decipiens* occurs mostly in Hokkaido Island in north Japan (Table 2). We also found that the fish species responsible for anisakidosis caused by *A. simplex* are different from those for *P. decipiens*, because the former is caused mostly by *Todarodes pacific*, *Thunnus thynnus*, and *Limanda herzenstieni* and the latter is caused mostly by *Theragra chalcogramma*, *Limanda herzenstieni*, *Cottus japonicus*, etc. (Table 3).

Table 2. Epidemiology: occurrence of anisakidosis—alteration of the parasite–host relationship of *Pseudoterranova decipiens*

1. *Pseudoterranova decipiens* found in anisakidosis patients in Hokkaido
2. Growth stage of anisakiosis and pseudoterranovosis found in the patient's stomach
3. Reported cases of anisakidosis caused by *Pseudoterranova decipiens* adult worms
4. From the host–parasite relationship to the parasite–host relationship

Table 3. Periodic variation of fish and squid that mediated anisakidosis in Japan

Species of infected fish and squid	1968	1974	1983	1996	
				A.[a]	P.[a]
Hippoglossus stenolepis		32	98	3	1
Todarodes pacific	1	29	77	12	1
Gadus macrocephalus		4	57	3	5
Thunnus thynnus	1	21	30	8	1
Paralichthys olivaceus	1	10	29	5	3
Scomber japonicus	4	18	19	3	
Fish of white meat		10		6	
Pleurogrammus azonus	2	3	6	2	
Limanda herzenstieni		2	6	1	
Oncorhynchus keta			1	7	1
Theragra chalcogramma	3	9			
Cottus japonicus		3		1	2
Podothecus sachi					2
Eleginus gracilis					2

[a] *A., Anasakis simplex*; *P., Pseudoterranova decipiens*.

Supporting this notion is the analysis of the infection rate of fish, which revealed that fish around Hokkaido, but not in the other islands of Japan, are infected with *P. decipiens* as well as *A. simplex* (Fig. 1). Anisakidosis is predominant in the southwestern area rather than in the north of Japan, because *Sardinops melanostictus* and *Scomber japonicus* are very commonly the fish responsible in the southwestern area in Japan. However, virtually no anisakidosis is caused by *P. decipiens* in the southwestern area of Japan because of a lack of fish infected with that species. Anisakidosis, caused both by *A. simplex* and *P. decipiens*, seems to occur predominantly in the winter season in Hokkaido, most likely because winter is the time when the fish responsible for this disease are caught.

Distribution of Intermediate and Final Hosts of Worms
Responsible for Anisakidosis

We next analyzed the infection rate of adult Anisakidae in the stomachs of sea mammals obtained off the coast of Hokkaido (Ishikura et al. 1996b).

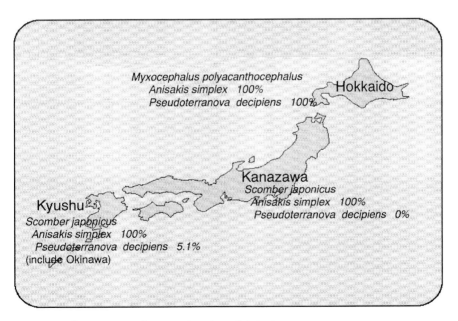

Fig. 1. Infection rates of intermediate host fish in the sea near Japan

The analysis revealed that *Callorhinus ursinus* migrating from the Sakhalin Islands are mostly infected with *P. decipiens* as well as with *A. simplex* (Fig. 2 and Table 4). Thus, the migration of *Callorhinus ursinus* from the Sakhalin and Aleutian Islands to the coast of Hokkaido seems to be responsible for the prevalence of anisakidosis caused by *P. decipiens* in Hokkaido (Ishikura et al. 1996b). Infection of fish with *A. simplex* in the southwestern area of Japan seemed to be attributable to sea mammals such as *Phocoena phocoena* in the tropical currents, which are never infected with *P. decipiens*. From these findings, we speculate that the incidence of anisakidosis and the pattern of infection of the worms responsible are dependent on the distribution of the intermediate and the final hosts of the Anisakidae species, which are in turn influenced by sea currents and climate.

Global Changes in Climate and Anisakidosis

In the Japan Sea, the distribution of both intermediate and final hosts can change the diversity and the density of anisakid nematodes in certain areas. Global climatic factors, such as acid rain, El Niño, and the ozone hole, may also change the local climate and currents. For example, El Niño, gives rise to problems such as unusual rainy seasons, a high incidence of typhoons, and cold summers in Japan. It can change the sea currents around Japan. Acid rain can change the plankton populations along the coasts. The ozone hole may change ground temperature and the distribution of plants and animals. Modern industrial society can also affect the ecosystem through industrial pollution in the form of dioxin emissions and the increase of CO_2 in the air, which factors are known to change the climate. All these climatic and environmental factors may cause alterations in the distribution of sea mammals, fish, and plankton, resulting in changes in the global and local incidence of anisakidosis (Ishikura et al. 1996b) (Fig. 3).

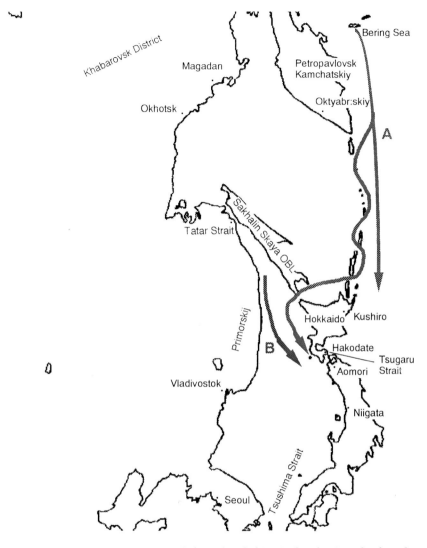

Fig. 2. Migration of marine mammals from their habitat in the Aleutian Islands to the coast of Hokkaido

Table 4. Number of Anisakidae parasitic in marine mammals

Species of marine mammals	No.	Species of worm[a]	Number of Anisakidae (approximate)
Phoca hispida	w-1	*A. simplex*	
Phoca vitulina	1	*A. simplex, P. decipiens*	5 000
	2	*A. simplex, P. decipiens*	90
	3	*A. simplex, P. decipiens*	100
	4	*A. simplex, P. decipiens*	50
	5	*P. decipiens*	150
	6	*A. simplex, P. decipiens*	50
	7	*A. simplex, P. decipiens*	50
	8	*P. decipiens*	75
	9	*A. simplex, C. osculatum*	80
Erignathus barbatus	1	*A. simplex, P. decipiens, C. osculatum*	3 000
Callorhinus ursinus	1	*A. simplex, P. decipiens, C. osculatum*	200
Eumetopias jubata	I-1	*P. decipiens*	270
	-2	*P. decipiens*	170
	-3	*P. decipiens*	250
	-4	*P. decipiens*	325
	-5	*P. decipiens adult*	7
	-6	*P. decipiens*	435
	-7	*P. decipiens*	275
	O-1	*A. simplex, P. decipiens, C. osculatum*	75
	-2	*P. decipiens*	450
	R-1	*P. decipiens*	450
	-2	*P. decipiens*	15 000
	-3	*P. decipiens*	15 000
	-4	*P. decipiens*	15 000
	O-3	*P. decipiens*	10 000
	-4	*P. decipiens*	10 000
	-5	*P. decipiens*	8 000
	-6	*P. decipiens*	15 000
	-7	*P. decipiens*	7 000
	-8	*A. simplex, P. decipiens, C. osculatum*	12 000
	-9	*A. simplex, P. decipiens, C. osculatum*	5 000
	R-5	*A. simplex, P. decipiens*	1 570
	-6	*A. simplex, P. decipiens*	126
	-9	*P. decipiens*	
	-10	*A. simplex, P. decipiens*	
	O-10	*A. simplex*	

[a] *A., Anisakis; P., Pseudoterranova; C., Contracaecum.*

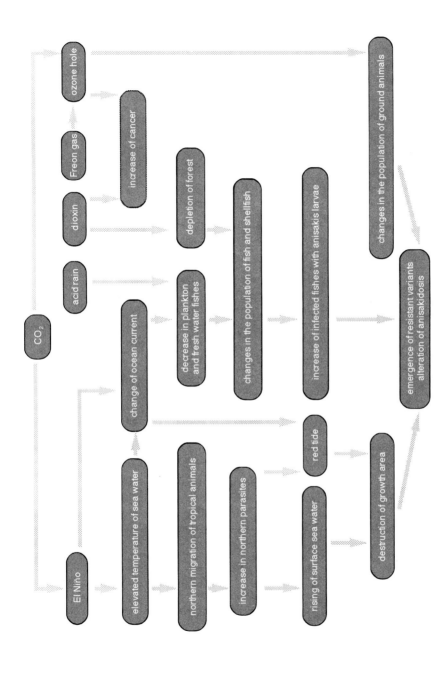

Fig. 3. The influence of environmental pollution on changes in Anisakidae

Conclusion

The unique incidence of anisakidosis caused by *Pseudoterranova decipiens* in Hokkaido was caused by fish infected with this anisakid worm that had migrated from the northern islands. Thus, it seems likely that global changes in climate may affect the population of those intermediate and final hosts of the anisakid species, resulting in the changed incidence of and variations in anisakidosis.

References

Ishikura H, Kikuchi K, Nagasawa K, Ooiwa T, Takamiya H, Sato N, Sugane K (1993) Anisakidae and anisakidosis. In: Tsieh S (ed) Progress in clinical parasitology. Springer-Verlag, Tokyo, pp 43–102

Takahashi S, Sato N, Ishikura H (1986) Establishment of monoclonal antibodies which discriminate the antigen distribution specifically found in *Anisakis* larvae C type I. J Parasitol 72:960–962

Takahashi S, Yagihashi A, Sato N, Kikuchi K (1990) Serodiagnosis of intestinal anisakiosis using micro-ELISA: diagnostic significance of patients' IgE. In: Ishikura H, Kikuchi K (eds) Intestinal anisakiosis in Japan. Springer-Verlag, Tokyo, pp 221–223

Yagihashi A, Sato N, Takahashi S, Ishikura H, Kikuchi K (1989) A serodiagnostic assay by microenzyme-linked immunosorbent assay for human anisakiosis using a monoclonal antibody specific for *Anisakis* larvae antigen. J Infect Dis 161:995–998

Ishikura H, Takahashi S, Ishikura H (1996a) Anisakidae and anisakidosis in Japan. In: Proceedings of the 2nd Japan-Korea Parasitologist's Seminar, April 2, 1996 Forum, Cheju 2, pp 50–63

Ishikura H, Takahashi S, Sato N, Matsuura A, Nitto H, Tsunokawa M, Kikuchi K (1996b) Epidemiology of anisakidosis and related human diseases and studies on parasites infecting marine mammals, fishes and squids. Bull Mar Biomed Inst Sapporo Med Univ 3:23–37

Ishikura H, Takahashi S, Sato N, Matsuura A, Kon S, Haysahi S, Nakamura K, Iino H, Kikuchi K (1997) Alteration of the outbreaks ratio between gastric and intestinal anisakiosis by using ELISA Kit of anti-*Anisakis* monoclonal antibody. Clin Parasitol 8:87–92

Takahashi S, Ishikura H, Kawai K, Hayashi S, Matsuura A, Kikuchi K (1997) Anisakidosis from the global point of view. Clin Parasitol 8:93–98

Nakamura K, Fujimoto T, Ishikura H, Takahashi S, Sato N, Matsurra A, Kon S, Kikuchi K (1997) Seroimmunodiagnosis of intestinal anisakidosis using micro plate method: evaluation of result from January 1995 to May 1997. Clin Parasitol 8:99–102

Takahashi S, Ishikura H, Sato N, Iwasa K (1993) Seroimmunodiagnostics of anisakiosis. In: Annual review of Immunology, 1993 (in Japanese). Chugai Igaku-Sha, Tokyo, pp. 212–217

Key Word Index